AF889099

Pathobiology

Journal of Immunopathology, Molecular and Cellular Biology

Founded 1938 as 'Schweizerische Zeitschrift für allgemeine Pathologie und Bakteriologie' by A. v. Albertini, A. Grumbach and H. Mooser, continued as 'Pathologia et Microbiologia' (1960–1975) and 'Experimental Cell Biology' (1976–1989); incorporating 'Pathology and Immunopathology Research', founded 1982 as 'Survey and Synthesis of Pathology Research' by J. Cruse and R.E. Lewis

KARGER

Printed in Switzerland
on acid-free paper by
Thür AG Offsetdruck, Pratteln

Appears bimonthly:
1 volume per year (6 issues)

Submission: Manuscripts should be addressed to:

Julius M. Cruse, MD, PhD
Department of Pathology
Immunopathology Section
University of Mississippi Medical Center
2500 North State Street
Jackson, MS 39216 (USA)

or to:

Mark I. Greene, MD, PhD
Director of Immunology
Department of Pathology
University of Pennsylvania
Philadelphia, PA 19104 (USA)

or to:

Dr. G.V. Sherbet
Cancer Research Unit
University of Newcastle upon Tyne
Medical School
Newcastle upon Tyne NE2 4HH (UK)

or to:

Prof. Dr. C. Sorg
Institut für Experimentelle Dermatologie
der Universität Münster
Von-Esmarch-Strasse 56
D-W-4400 Münster (FRG)

Manuscripts should be submitted in triplicate (with three sets of illustrations of which one is an original), typewritten double-spaced on one side of the paper, with a wide margin.

Conditions: Manuscripts must be written in English, and are all subject to editorial review. Manuscripts are received with the explicit understanding that they are not submitted for simultaneous consideration by any other publication. Submission of an article for publication implies the transfer of the copyright from the author to the publisher upon acceptance. Accepted papers become the permanent property of 'Pathobiology' and may not be reproduced by any means, in whole or in part, without the written consent of the publisher. It is the author's responsibility to obtain permission to reproduce illustrations, tables, etc. from other publications.

Arrangement

Title page: The first page of each paper should indicate the title (main title underlined), the authors' names, and the institute where the work was conducted. A short title for use as running head as well as the full address of the author to whom correspondence should be sent are also required.

Full address: The exact postal address complete with postal code must be given at the bottom of the title page. Please also supply phone and fax numbers.

Key words: For indexing purposes, a list of 3–10 key words in English is essential

Abstract: Each paper needs an abstract of up to 10 lines.

Small type: Paragraphs which can or must be set in smaller type (case histories, test methods, etc.) should be indicated with a 'p' (petit) in the margin on the left-hand side.

Footnotes: Avoid footnotes. When essential, they are numbered consecutively and typed at the foot of the appropriate page.

Tables and illustrations: Tables and illustrations (both numbered in Arabic numerals) should be prepared on separate sheets. Tables require a heading and figures a legend, also prepared on a separate sheet. For the reproduction of illustrations, only good drawings and original photographs can be accepted; negatives or photocopies cannot be used. When possible, group several illustrations on one block for reproduction (max. size 181 × 223 mm) or provide crop marks. On the back of each illustration, indicate its number, the author's name, and 'top'. Color illustrations are reproduced at the author's expense.

References: In the text identify references by Arabic numerals [in square brackets]. Material submitted for publication but not yet accepted should be noted as 'unpublished data' and not be included in the reference list. The list of references should include only those publications which are cited in the text. Do not alphabetize; number references in the order in which they are first mentioned in the text. The surnames of the authors followed by initials should be given. There should be no punctuation other than a comma to separate the authors. Cite all authors, 'et al' is not sufficient. Abbreviate journal names according to the Index Medicus system. (Also see International Committee of Medical Journal Editors: Uniform requirements for manuscripts submitted to biomedical journals. Br Med J 1988;296:401–405.)

Examples

(a) Papers published in periodicals: Kauffman HF, van der Heide S, Beaumont F, Blok H, de Vries K: Class-specific antibody determination against *Aspergillus fumigatus* by means of the enzyme-linked immunosorbent assay. III. Comparative study: IgG, IgA, IgM ELISA titers, precipitating antibodies and IgE binding after fractionation of the antigen. Int Arch Allergy Appl Immunol 1986;80:-300–306.

(b) Monographs: Matthews DE, Farewell VT: Using and Understanding Medical Statistics. Basel, Karger, 1985.

(c) Edited books: Hardy WD Jr, Essex M: FeLV-induced feline acquired immune deficiency syndrome: A model for human AIDS; in Klein E (ed): Acquired Immunodeficiency Syndrome. Prog Allergy. Basel, Karger, 1986, vol 37, pp 353–376.

Further details: Authors may consult our leaflet 'Rules for the Preparation of Manuscripts', available on request from the Publisher, S. Karger AG, P.O. Box, CH–4009 Basel (Switzerland).

Page charges: Page charges may be levied if the allotted size of the manuscript, as stipulated by the editors of the journal, is exceeded. Each additional complete or partial page is charged to the author at SFr. 225.–/US$ 150.00. 3 manuscript pages (including tables, illustrations and references) are equal to approximately one printed page.

Galley proofs: Unless indicated otherwise, galley proofs are sent to the first-named author and should be returned with the least possible delay. Alterations made in galley proofs, other than the correction of printer's errors, are charged to the author. No page proofs are supplied.

Reprints: Order forms and a price list are sent with the galley proofs. Orders submitted after the issue is printed are subject to considerably higher prices. Allow five weeks from date of publication for delivery of reprints.

KARG

Pathobiology

Publication data: Volume 60, 1992 of 'Pathobiology' appears with 6 issues.
Subscription rates: Subscriptions run for a full calendar year. Prices are given per volume, surface postage included.
Personal subscription:
SFr. 202.80, US$ 135.30.
(Must be in the name of, billed to, and paid by an individual. Order must be marked 'personal subscription'.)
Institutional subscription:
(Regular rate.) SFr. 676.–, US$ 451.00.
Members of the AAI: SFr. 270.40, US$ 180.40.
Airmail postage: SFr. 35.–, US$ 30.00.
(Extra per volume.)
Microform subscription:
SFr. 338.–, US$ 225.50.
(Available exclusively to subscribers of the paper edition.)
Single issues and back volumes: Information on availability and prices can be obtained through the Publisher.
Advertising: Correspondence and rate requests should be addressed to the Publisher.

Subscription orders: Orders can be placed at agencies, bookstores, directly with the Publisher S. Karger AG, P.O. Box, CH – 4009 Basel (Switzerland) or with any of the following distributors:
Deutschland:
S. Karger GmbH, Lörracher Strasse 16A
Postfach, D-W-7800 Freiburg
France: Librairie Luginbühl
36, bd de Latour-Maubourg, F-75007 Paris
Great Britain, Ireland:
S. Karger Publishers, 11 Ravenscroft Road
Beckenham, Kent BR3 4TP
USA: S. Karger Publishers, Inc.
26 West Avon Road, P.O. Box 529
Farmington, CT 06085
India, Bangladesh, Sri Lanka:
S. Karger India Subscription Agency
B – 5/132 Safdarjung Enclave
New Delhi-110029
Japan: Katakura Libri, Inc.
36-9 Hongo 3-chome, Bunkyo-ku, Tokyo 113
Change of address: Both old and new address should be stated and sent to the subscription source.

Bibliographic indices: This journal is regularly listed in bibliographic services, including *Current Contents®*.

KARGER

The Macrophage

The Macrophage 1992

Abstracts

Organized under the Patronage of the Upper Rhine Universities

European Conference on Basic and Clinical Aspects of Macrophage Biology
Regensburg, FRG
September 20–22, 1992

Guest Editor
Reinhard Andreesen, Regensburg

KARGER

Pathobiology

Vol. 60, Supplement 1, 1992

Acknowledgement for Support

Major Sponsors

Asta Pharma
Baxter
Bayer AG
Boehringer Mannheim
Essex Pharma
Dr. Falk Pharma GmbH
Hoffmann-La Roche AG
ICI Pharma
Sandoz AG
Tropon GmbH

Contributors

Beckmann
H. Biermann GmbH
Biotest Pharma
Boehringer Ingelheim
Ciba-Geigy AG
E. Merck KG
Marion Merrell Dow GmbH
Pfizer GmbH
S. Karger AG, Basel
Glaxo

S. Karger
Medical and Scientific Publishers
Basel · Freiburg · Paris · London
New York · New Delhi · Bangkok
Singapore · Tokyo · Sydney

Drug Dosage
The authors and the publisher have exerted every effort to ensure that drug selection and dosage set forth in this text are in accord with current recommendations and practice at the time of publication. However, in view of ongoing research, changes in government regulations, and the constant flow of information relating to drug therapy and drug reactions, the reader is urged to check the package insert for each drug for any change in indications and dosage and for added warnings and precautions. This is particularly important when the recommended agent is a new and/or infrequently employed drug.

Printed in Switzerland on acid-free paper by
Reinhardt Druck, Basel
ISBN 3-8055-5689-6

Contents

Organizing Committee

Location

Universität Regensburg
Klinikum
Franz-Josef-Strauss Allee 11
D-W-8400 Regensburg

Scientific Committee

R. Andreesen, Regensburg (Chair)
J. Ciesielski-Treska, Strasbourg
J. van Damme, Leuven
J. Bartholeyns, Paris
J. Bendtzen, Copenhagen
E. Ferber, Freiburg
G. Figdor, Amsterdam
M. Freudenberg, Freiburg
C. Galanos, Freiburg
G. Garotta, Basel
D. Gemsa, Marburg
S. Gordon, Oxford
R. Landmann, Basel
J. Lazdins, Basel
H.G. Leser, Regensburg
D. Männel, Regensburg
A. Mantovani, Milano
J. Mauel, Lausanne
M. Parant, Paris
P. Poindron, Strasbourg
H.J. Radzun, Kiel
C. Sorg, Münster

Organization

K.J. Bross
A. Droll
R. Eckert
B. Hemmerich
B. Hennemann
S. Krause
M. Kreutz
A. Rehm
A. Reichle
M. Reng

Scientific Program

	Sunday, September 20
15.00	Registration and Poster Mounting
17.20–19.30	Plenary Session Macrophages and Inflammation
19.30	Welcome Reception
	Monday, September 21
8.30–10.30	Plenary Session Macrophage Activation and Cytotoxicity
11.00–13.00	Plenary Session Macrophages and Cell Interaction
14.00–17.00	Poster Session
	Tuesday, September 22
8.30–10.30	Plenary Session Macrophage Ontogeny and Heterogeneity
11.00–13.00	Plenary Session Macrophages and Infection
14.00–16.00	Plenary Session Macrophages and Disease

Sunday, September 20

15.00	Registration and Poster Mounting
17.00	Welcome by Prof. Dr. R. Andreesen, Conference Chairman Prof. Dr. J. Sauer, Vice President of the University of Regensburg
	HIV-Induced Syncytia Formation in Human Macrophages – A Microcinematographic Study Von Briesen H, Sander U, Seack KH, Kreutz M, Becker K, Müller S, Rübsamen-Waigmann H, Andreesen R (Frankfurt, Regensburg)
17.20–19.30	**Plenary Session Macrophages and Inflammation** (*Chairpersons:* M. Parant, C. Galanos)
	Soluble Cytokine Receptors and the Treatment of Inflammation Urdal D (Seattle)
	Genetic Accessibility and Endotoxin Responsiveness of the TNF Locus in Macrophages, Fibroblasts and Hybrid Cells Beutler B, Kruvs Y, Harter N (Dallas)
	Autoantibodies to Macrophage Hormones (Cytokines) – Detection and Biological Significance Bendtzen K, Hansen MB, Diamant M, Svenson M (Copenhagen)
	Structural and Functional Identification of two Human, Tumor-Derived Monocyte Chemotactic Proteins Belonging to the Chemokine Family Van Damme J, Proost P, Lenaerts JP, Opdenakker G (Leuven)
	Lipid A Partial Structures: Inhibition of LPS-Induced Monokine Production Ulmer AJ, Feist W, Kirikae T, Kirikae F, Heine H, Kusumoto S, Kusama T, Brade H, Schade U, Rietschel Th, Flad HD (Borstel)
19.30	Welcome Reception in front of the Lecture Theatre

Monday, September 21

8.30–10.30	**Plenary Session Macrophage Activation and Cytotoxicity** (*Chairpersons:* G. Garotta, D. Gemsa)
	Cytokine Induced Synthesis from L-Arginine: Implications from Cell-Mediated Immunity Hibbs JB jr. (Salt Lake City)
	NF-KB: A Transcriptional Activator and Coordinator of Immediate-Early Gene Expression in Macrophages Baeuerle PA, Schreck R, Müller J, Ziegler-Heitbrock L (Munich)
	Activation of Iron Responsive Element Binding Protein by 7,8-Dihydroneopterin in Human Monocytic Cells Weiss G, Doppler W, Hentze MW, Werner-Felmayer G, Fuchs D, Wachter H (Innsbruck)
	Zymosan-Induced Tyrosine Phosphorylations in Human Monocytes: Role of Protein Kinase C Sanguedolce MV, Capo C, Bouhamdan M, Bongrand Pierre, Huang CK, Mege JL (Marseille)
	Antagonistic Effects between Endogenous Interferon-B and Interleukin 4 in Mouse Macrophages Zawatzky R, Nickolaus P, Falk W (Heidelberg)
	Effect of LPS on Membrane CD14 in Human Monocytes and Macrophages Landmann R, Galanos C, Zimmerli W (Basel)
10.30	Coffee Break

11.00–13.00	**Plenary Session Macrophages and Cell Interaction** (*Chairpersons:* D. Männel, J. Lazdins)
	The Role of Integrins in Macrophage Biology Hogg N (London)
	Identification of Macrophage Adhesion Molecules by Monoclonal Antibody Strategy Fraser I, Hughes D, Gordon S (Oxford)
	Effects of IL-10 on Human Monocyte Function Figdor CG, De Waal Malefijt R, Te Velde AA, De Vries JE (Amsterdam)
	Production of a Novel Soluble Mediator during the Interaction of T_h1-Lymphocytes and Bone Marrow-Derived Macrophages Cultured in GM-CSF Germann T, Rüde E (Mainz)
	Apoptosis in TNF-Alpha Dependent Monocyte Mediated Leukemic Cell Death. A Morphological, Functional and Flow Cytometric Analysis Van De Loosdrecht AA, Ossenkoppele GJ, Beelen RHJ, Broekhoven MG, Langenhuijsen MMAC (Amsterdam)
	Modulation of Monokine Production by themselves or by Xenobiotics Parant MA (Paris)
13.00–14.00	Lunch
14.00–17.00	**Poster Session** General Poster Viewing 14.00–15.00 Poster Presentation; authors are requested to be present at their posters: 15.00–16.00 for posters with even numbers 16.00–17.00 for posters with uneven numbers
17.30	Boat ride on the danube
	Tuesday, September 22
8.30–10.30	**Plenary Session Macrophage Ontogeny and Heterogeneity** (*Chairpersons:* P. Poindron, C. Sorg)
	Cytokine Interactions in the Growth of Myeloid Precursor Cells Fibbe WE, Kluin-Nelemans JC, Falkenburg JHF, Willemze R (Leiden)
	Macrophage Differentiation in Macrophage Colony Stimulating Factor-Deficient Mice for the Osteopetrotic (OP) Mutation Takahashi K, Naito M, Morioka Y, Umeda S, Shultz LD (Kumamoto)
	Phenotypic and Functional Characterization of $CD64^+$ Monocytes, a Minor Human Monocyte Subpopulation with High Antigen-Presenting Capacity Grage-Griebenow E, Lorenzen D, Flad HD, Ernst M (Borstel)
	Cloning and Expression of a Human Monocyte/Macrophage Antigen Detected by the Monoclonal Antibody Ki-M1P Lilischkis R, Salmassi A, Zschunke F, Heidorn K, Jaquet K, Heidebrecht H, Kreipe H, Parwaresch MR, Radzun HJ (Kiel, Göttingen)
	Regulation of TNF-Alpha-mRNA Synthesis in Kupffer Cells in the LPS-Perfused Rat Liver: A Non-Radioactive in situ Hybridization Study Hoffmann R, Grewe M, Estler HC, Schulze-Specking A, Decker K (Freiburg)
	Functional and Receptor Characterization of Mouse Peritoneal Macrophages Plasman N, Vray B (Bruxelles)
	Comparative Interaction of Glycated and Oxidized Low Density Lipoproteins with Human Monocyte-Derived Macrophages Gugliucci Creriche A, Siffert JC, Dumont S, Stahl AJC (Strasbourg)
10.30	Coffee Break

11.00–13.00 **Plenary Session Macrophages and Infection**
(*Chairpersons:* M. Freudenberg, J. Bartholeyns)

The Role of Microglia Cells in Viral Infections
Brinkmann R, Sedgwick J, Schwender S, Imrich H, Dörries R, Ter Meulen V (Würzburg)

Biochemical Mechanism(s) of the Macrophage Response to Bacterial Lipopolysaccharide
Kirikae T, Zhang X, Kirikae F, Lei MG, Morrison DC (Kansas City)

The Macrophage Response to Bacteria and Bacterial Products
Keller R (Zürich)

Purification and Characterization of Murine LPS Binding Protein
Gallay P, Glauser MP, Barras C, Ulevitch RJ, Tobias PS, Baumgartner JD, Heumann D (Zürich, La Jolla)

Differential Induction of Macrophage Early Genes, C-FOS, KC, JE and TNF-Alpha by Lipoarabinomannan from Avirulent and Virulent Strains of Mycobacterium Tuberculosis
Roach TIA, Chatterjeed, Blackwell JM (Cambridge)

Molecular Pathogenesis of Monocytes/Macrophages HIV-1 Infection
Raoul H, Le Naour R, Mabondzo A, Boussin F, Dormont D (Fontenay aux Roses)

13.00–14.00 Lunch

14.00–16.00 **Plenary Session Macrophages and Disease**
(*Chairpersons:* A. Mantovani, R. Andreesen)

The Role of Mononuclear Phagocytes in the Pathogenesis of Atherosclerosis
Schmitz G, Kovacs E, Rothe G (Regensburg)

Effect of Soluble MoIFN-Gamma-R Treatment on the Development of Spontaneous Autoimmune Disease in NZB/W F1 Mice
Ozmen L, Ryffel B, Fountoulakis M, Gentz R, Garotta G (Basel)

The Role of Macrophages in Experimental Lyme Borreliosis
Modolell M, Schaible U, Corraliza I, Rittig M, Simon M (Freiburg)

Myelin P2 Protein Induces Proinflammatory Cytokines mRNA Accumulation and Secretion by Human Cultured Phagocytes
Baron P, Constantin G, Cassatella MA (Verona)

RM3/1 Surface Expression on Monocytes is Directly Correlated to Glucocorticoid Receptor Binding Affinity
Erpenstein U, Rohdewald P, Sorg C (Münster)

Encapsulation of Tissue for Transplantation Does not Protect from Macrophage Mediated Lysis via Nitric Oxide in in vitro Experiments
Kröncke KD, Wiegand F, Kolb-Bachofen V (Düsseldorf)

The Role of Tumor Necrosis Factor in an Experimental Metastasis Model
Orosz P, Echtenacher B, Männel DN (Heidelberg, Regensburg)

Poster Session

Macrophages and Inflammation

1 A Receptor for C-Reactive Protein, Isolated and Purified from Rat Macrophages
Alsdorff K, Kolb-Bachofen V

2 Effect of Protein Kinase Inhibitors on Tannin-Mediated Arachidonic Acid Release from Rabbit Alveolar Macrophages
Desrues B, Rohrbach MS

Macrophage Activation and Cytotoxicity

Macrophages and Infection

Macrophages and Disease

Pathobiology 1992;60(suppl 1):1–38

Abstracts

LUMINOL-DEPENDENT CHEMILUMINESCENCE OF MONOCYTES, BUT NOT OF NEUTROPHILS, DEPENDS ENTIRELY ON THE TRIGGER-MEDIATED EXTRACELLULAR DEPLOYMENT OF CELL-DERIVED MYELOPEROXIDASE AND REACTIVE OXYGEN SPECIES.

Daniel Albrecht and Thomas W. Jungi, Institute of Veterinary Virology, University of Berne, Länggass-Str. 122, CH-3012 Berne, Switzerland.

Luminol-enhanced chemiluminescence is an often-used method to demonstrate and quantitate an oxidative burst. It is more sensitive than measurement of superoxide-inhibitable cytochrome C reduction. Its drawback, however, is its dependency on several metabolic events. It is dependent on both superoxide generation, and myeloperoxidase activity. Furthermore, it has been shown that both intracellular and extracellular events are measured. This complexity precludes the use of the method for studying biological response modification, since modulatory effects may affect any of the diverse parameters contributing to luminol-enhanced chemiluminescence (LCL). We have used LCL to monitor for signal transduction in monocytes by antibody crosslinking of either surface constituents or of cell receptor-associated ligands. We now have analysed the metabolic events leading to LCL and provide evidence that in monocytes, LCL is an entirely extracellular event requiring both the release of myeloperoxidase, and the generation of superoxide. This is in contrast to LCL of neutrophils which has both an intracellular and an extracellular component. The advent of adding H_2O_2 to the assay allows to measure the degranulation-dependent moiety separately. As described earlier, LCL in the presence of horse radish peroxidase and azide represents extracellular H_2O_2 generation mediated by an NADPH-dependent oxidase. Using these modified LCL systems, modulation of either event can now be measured independently. Moreover, the former procedure allows to study degranulation kinetically and to investigate signal transduction cascades leading to degranulation and/or frustrated phagocytosis.

A RECEPTOR FOR C-REACTIVE PROTEIN (CRP), ISOLATED AND PURIFIED FROM RAT MACROPHAGES

Kathrin Alsdorff and Victoria Kolb-Bachofen

Institute for Immunobiology, Fac. of Medicine. Heinrich-Heine-University, DÜSSELDORF, Germany.

Rat Kupffer cells are able to endocytose particulate ligands via a galactose-specific binding activity. We could recently show, that this "particle receptor" is identical to a membrane-associated form of the well known acute phase protein C-reactive protein (CRP). This CRP is a peripheral membrane protein attached to a hypothetical membrane receptor in a Ca^{2+}-dependent way. We now have used a new method , the "gold affinity chromatography", to isolate and purify this receptor from isolated rat Kupffer cells.

Freshly isolated rat Kupffer cells were incubated with galactosylated bovine serum albumin adsorbed onto colloidal gold particles as a specific ligand for membrane associated CRP. By lysing the cells with detergent, several centrifugation steps and separation from the gold-labelled ligand by adding EDTA, we obtained a receptor protein preparation.

For purification we used rat CRP also adsorbed onto colloidal gold as a direct ligand for the receptor protein. As described for the isolation, the receptor was separated from the ligand by EDTA after centrifugation. In an SDS gel the enriched CRP receptor protein consisted of two bands with relative molecular weights of 59 and 61 kDa.

From peritoneal macrophages the receptor protein could also be isolated and purified by treating the cells similar as described for the Kupffer cells.

In conclusion, rat Kupffer cells and peritoneal macrophages express a membrane receptor for CRP. Future investigations will have to show, whether all macrophage subpopulations possess this receptor protein.

1015–2008/92/0607–0001
$2.75/0

MEASUREMENT OF TNFA MRNA PRODUCTION OF MONONUCLEAR CELLS ISOLATED FROM MUCOSAL BIOPSIES BY QUANTITATIVE RNA-POLYMERASE CHAIN REACTION.

T. Andus, S.R. Targan*, R. Deem*, J. Schölmerich, H. Toyoda+.

Medizinische Klinik der Universität Regensburg I, *UCLA and +Cedars-Sinai Medical Center, Los Angeles, CA 90048

Increased numbers of activated macrophages in the mucosa are a characteristic feature in inflamed lesions of patients with inflammatory bowel disease. Activated mononuclear lamina propria cells produce tumor necrosis factor α (TNFα), which has been shown to kill human epithelial targets such as HT-29. Therefore, we examined the role of TNFα in the in situ inflammatory process using mucosal biopsies. Because only a small number of cells can be obtained from biopsies, we developed a method to measure TNFα-mRNA by quantitative polymerase chain reaction (PCR). TNFα message was quantitated by co-reveres transcription and co-amplification of cellular RNA with an artificial TNFα-RNA containing an internal deletion after reverse transcription. Using our quantitative PCR method we detected measurable TNFα RNA in as few as 10^4 lamina propria mononuclear cells. The level of TNFα message was approximately 8 fold increased in cells from inflammatory lesions of CD patients compared to normal mucosa. In conclusion quantitative PCR allows the measurement of mRNA concentrations of cytokines in mucosal lesions and the study of the regulation of cytokine mRNAs in mononuclear cells isolated from mucosal biopsies.

INDUCTION OF TNF-α SECRETION BY MURAMYL DIPEPTIDE CONJUGATED TO AN ANTI-MACROPHAGE MONOCLONAL ANTIBODY,

by Régine AUDRAN[a], Patrick MIDOUX[b], Annie-Claude ROCHE[b], Michel MONSIGNY[b] and Louis TOUJAS[a].
([a]: Département de Biologie, Centre Régional de Lutte contre le Cancer, BP 6279, 35062 Rennes-cedex, France and [b]: Département de Biochimie des glycoconjugués et lectines endogènes, Centre de Biophysique moléculaire, CNRS, INSERM et Université, 1, rue Haute, 45071 Orléans-cedex 02, France).

Muramyl dipeptide (MDP) targetted with an anti-macrophage monoclonal antibody (MAb) might be used as a cancer treatment. This hypothesis was first investigated using a mouse experimental model. A rat anti-mouse Mac-1 MAb (MAb 3A33) was radiolabelled, injected intravenously into mice and found to bind to macrophages and to segregate predominantly in inflammatory foci and tumor grafts. (Collet et al, Cancer Immunol. Immunother., 1988, 26, 237-242). MAb 3A33 was next substituted with 5 molecules of a neutral polypeptide (partially gluconoylated poly-L-lysine) bearing 15 MDP moieties forming MAb 3A33 -(-SS-,$GlcA_{180}$-, MDP_{15} -PLK)5 complexes. This conjugate induced cytotoxicity of mouse peritoneal macrophages, and was more efficient than the various relevant controls (Midoux et al. Bioconjugate Chem., 1992, 3, 194-199). Recently, a similar compound was prepared using a mouse anti-human CD11b MAb (kindly given by Immunotech) as a vector. Anti-CD11b MAb-(-SS-, $GlcA_{65}$-,MDP_{30}-PLK)2 conjugate was tested for its ability to induce TNF-α secretion in cultured human monocytes. TNF-α was assayed with a cytotoxicity test using actinomycin D-treated L929 cells. Monocytes obtained from blood mononuclear cells were left to adhere for 8 hours, to allow spontaneous TNF-α release to be completed, before adding MDP-conjugates. Anti-CD11b MAb-MDP conjugate induced the secretion of a cytotoxic factor, the activity of which was abolished by anti-TNF-α antibody. In control experiments using unspecific antibody-MDP conjugates, no such factor could be detected. Taken together, the present results suggest that the antitumor activity of monocyte-macrophage might be stimulated in vivo by MDP vectorized by specific antibodies.

INFLUENZA A VIRUS INFECTION OF MACROPHAGES: INDUCTION OF TWO DIFFERENT TYPES OF TNF-α mRNA

M.Bacher, H.Sprenger, A.Bender, A.Rischkowsky, M.Nain and D.Gemsa

Institute of Immunology, Philipps University, Marburg, Germany

Infection of murine PU5-1.8 macrophages and human monocytes by influenza A virus, strain Puerto Rico 8 (H1N1), is associated with release of tumor necrosis factor-α (TNF-α) and other cytokines. On a molecular level, Northern blot analysis detected a massive TNF-α mRNA accumulation which consisted of a regular and an additional, high molecular weight (hmw) mRNA species. In this study we were interested in characterizing hmw TNF-α mRNA. We found that hmw TNF-α mRNA could be detected by plasmid-derived as well as by PCR-amplified, exon-specific cDNA probes. The presence of genomic intron sequences, which characterize a primary TNF-α mRNA transcript, was ruled out by failure to hybridize with intron-specific TNF-α cDNA probes. Several other possibilities were taken into consideration: the two TNF-α mRNA species may be generated by alternative splicing or may deviate in different 3' and 5'ends. With the use of rapid amplification of cDNA ends (RACE) we amplified regions between defined single point transcripts and 3' or 5'ends. Extension of cDNAs from the end of the message to specific primer sequences was accomplished by primers annealing to the natural 3'end or synthetically prolonged poly A 3' tails. Whereas the 3'RACE showed no difference between PCR-amplified 3'cDNA ends of regular and hmw TNF-α mRNA, additional hmw products were detected during the 5'RACE. These findings demonstrate that upon influenza A virus infection of macrophages, a 5'end-elongated TNF-α mRNA was generated which will be further characterized with respect to base pair sequence and possible biological activity.

NF-KB: A TRANSCRIPTIONAL ACTIVATOR AND COORDINATOR OF IMMEDIATE-EARLY GENE EXPRESSION IN MACROPHAGES

Patrick A. Baeuerle, Ralf Schreck, Judith Müller and Löms Ziegler-Heitbrock[1]
Gene Center, Ludwig-Maximilians-University Munich, Am Klopferspitz 18a, D-8033 Martinsried, and [1]Institute for Immunology, Goethestr. 31, D-8000 Munich, Germany.

Activation of macrophages, for instance, in response to lipopolysaccharide (LPS) and TNF, leads to a rapid and coordinate induction of many genes encoding cytokines and other effector molecules of the inflammatory response. The coordinate induction of a group of these genes appears to be achieved by the use of the same inducible transcriptional activator. There is evidence that nuclear factor kappa B (NF-κB) is involved in the induction of the genes encoding TNF-α, IL-1, Il-6, IL-8, G-CSF, GM-CSF, M-CSF, IL-3, tissue factor and IL-2R α-chain. All these genes contain in enhancer elements functional binding sites for NF-kB cooperating with other factor binding sites in gene induction.

NF-κB is an inducible transcription factor that is activated when many different cell types are exposed to TNF, IL-1, LPS, viruses, UV light, γ rays and mild oxidative stress. A hallmark of NF-κB is that, in non-stimulated cells, it resides in the cytoplasm in complex with the inhibitory subunit IκB. Stimulation of cells results in release of IκB, nuclear transport of NF-κB and finally binding of NF-κB to promoter and enhancer elements in genes -- an event causing the initiation of mRNA synthesis from genes.

TNF is known to induce the production of superoxide and H_2O_2 in cells. This prompted us to test whether H_2O_2 itself is capapble of inducing NF-κB. Micromolar concentrations of H_2O_2 could indeed potently activate NF-κB in a human T cell line and the activation was blocked by N-acetyl-L-cysteine (NAC), dithiocarbamates and non-sulfur iron/copper chelators. This shows that NF-κB is an oxidative stress-responsive factor. Various antioxidants also blocked induction of NF-κB by LPS and TNF in macrophages/monocytes. These results suggest that reactive oxygen intermediates play a role as messengers or modulators in the activation of NF-κB by LPS and other agents. Antioxidants (NAC etc.) may thus turn out as pharmceutics with the potential to suppress activation of NF-κB and, thereby, activation of macrophages and monocytes.

NITRIC OXIDE (NO) PRODUCTION BY SPLENIC MACROPHAGES IS RESPONSIBLE FOR THE DEPRESSION OF LYMPHOPROLIFERATIVE RESPONSES OBSERVED AFTER BURN INJURY IN RATS.

T. Bamberger*, J. Mathieu**, I. Masson*,.M. De Sousa*, B. Chanaud, S. Strzalko*, L. Chauvelot-Moachon, J.P. Giroud and I. Florentin.

*Département de Pharmacologie (URA CNRS 595), Hôpital Cochin, Paris. **Département de Radiobiochimie, Centre de Recherche du Service de Santé des Armées, La Tronche, France.

Impairement of cell-mediated immunity develops early after burn injury and likely is at the origin of frequent septic complications. T suppressor cells and low molecular weight suppressor factors, including prostaglandin E2, have been implicated. We show that the defective lymphoproliferative responses to T cell mitogens (PHA and Con A) observed after thermal injury in rats can be restored by macrophage depletion (adherence) of spleen cells or by the action of chloroadenosine which is toxic for macrophages (Masson et al, abstract in the same issue). In the present work, we investigate whether nitric oxide (NO) could be the mediator of macrophage suppressive activity .

In the first part of this work, we demonstrated that the NO donors, molsidomine and sodium nitroprusside, inhibited, in a dose dependent manner, the proliferative responses to T cell mitogens of normal spleen cells from Wistar rats. Spleen cells from some rats responded poorly to mitogens. The addition to the cultures of inhibitors of the NO synthase, (N^G-monomethyl-L-arginine, N-nitro-L-arginine methyl ester and L- canavanine) allowed the increase of the responses to the level of high responder rats.

Lymphoproliferative responses are strongly depressed 3-4 days after thermal injury. They are fully restored when spleen cells are cultured in presence of NO synthase inhibitors. In parallel, NO release was measured (by dosage of nitrites with the Griess reagent) in the supernatants of spleen cells stimulated with Con A. We observed a correlation between impaired responses to mitogens and increased production of NO.

These results demonstrate that in rats, NO is an immunosupressive agent that is responsible for impaired lymphocyte reactivity to mitogens in normal and pathological situations.

Activated microglia in vivo rapidly synthesize Alzheimer βA4-amyloid precursor protein (APP)

R.B. Banati*, J. Gehrmann*, C. Czech, U. Mönning, L. L. Jones, G. König, K. Beyreuther and G.W. Kreutzberg*

*Department of Neuromorphology, Max-Planck-Institute of Psychiatry, D-8033 Martinsried near Munich; Center for Molecular Biology Heidelberg (ZMBH), University of Heidelberg, Im Neuenheimer Feld 282, D-6900 Heidelberg, Federal Republic of Germany.

Upon acute activation microglia, the immuneffector cells of the brain parenchyma express the amyloid precursor protein (APP) that is otherwise prominent in pathological structures related to Alzheimer's disease. In this disease complex amyloid-bearing neuritic plaques contain βA4-amyloid protein, the amyloid precursor protein (APP) and inflammatory proteins. The accompanying activation of microglia has mostly been viewed as a secondary reaction to amyloid deposits.

Activation of microglia was performed in a graded fashion. Transection of peripheral nerves such as the facial or sciatic nerve causes a microglial reaction within hours in the nucleus of origin or in projection areas of the CNS. A predominantly glial up-regulation of APP mRNA and protein could be detected as early as 6 h post lesion not only at the site of affected neuronal cell bodies but also in corresponding projection areas. Its time course suggests rapid transneuronal signalling to glial cells in the projection area. Light and electron microscopy demonstrate that microglia, which are cells of mononuclear phagocyte lineage and comprise up to 20% of all glial cells, are the dominant source for non-neuronal APP-expression. Ultrastructurally, brain perivascular cells within the basal lamina constitutively express APP and thus are a possible source of vascular amyloid.

Microglia express leukocyte-derived L-APP mRNA and protein that have recently been described in mononuclear cells of the immune system. Increased L-APP-expression may serve as a potential marker for glial/microglial activation. Such immune-mediated amyloidogenesis initiated by microglia might have implications for the treatment of neurodegenerative diseases.

CELLULAR COMPOSITION IN THE PERITONEAL CAVITY AND CYTOTOXIC FUNCTION OF PERITONEAL MACROPHAGES FROM PATIENTS WITH OVARIAN CANCER; EFFECT OF TUMOR NECROSIS FACTOR-α TREATMENT IN VIVO.

R.H.J. Beelen, C.D. Richters, A.A. van de Loosdrecht[2], C.W. Burger[1], G.J.M. Eppink, A.C. van Hof[1], P. Kenemans[1].

Dept. of Cell Biology, Obstetrics and Gynaecology[1] and Haematology[2], Free University Hospital and Faculty of Medicine, Vrije Universiteit, Amsterdam, The Netherlands

In patients with epithelial ovarian cancer (EOC), the cellular composition in the peritoneal cavity and the functional capacities of the peritoneal cells (PC) are unknown. Especially the peritoneal macrophages (mϕ) could play an important role in defense against tumour cells. To study the cellular compostition in the peritoneal cavity and the functional capacities of PC, these cells were obtained from three patients with EOC. The PC were immunophenotyped and tested functionally *in vitro* in a cytotoxicity assay (method see van de Loosdrecht et al, this symposium). PC from healthy women undergoing laparoscopic sterilization served as controls. Furthermore, one of the patients was treated with a single dose of 0.1 mg tumour necrosis factor-α (TNF-α), intraperitoneally administered. PC were obtained after 24 hours, after 1 week and before the treatment.
Our results show that ovariumcarcinoma patients have a lower percentage of macrophages (mϕ) in the peritoneal cavity than healthy persons. Peritoneal mϕ of patients were less capable of killing U 937 tumour cells as compared to control peritoneal mϕ. However, in the TNF-α treated patient the cytotoxic capacities of the peritoneal mϕ were strongly improved increasing from 17% to 80% at an E/T ratio of 10. Thus, the peritoneal mϕ in this patient were activated *in vivo* to a tumouricidal state. The lower percentage peritoneal mϕ and the impaired function of these cells from patients with ovarian cancer is probably due to the disease or previous treatment.

ISOLATION AND CHARACTERISATION OF ANTIGEN PRESENTING CELLS FROM THE HUMAN PERITONEAL CAVITY.

M.G.H. Betjes, C.W. Tuk, * D.G. Struijk, R.H.J. Beelen.
Dept. Cell biology, Vrije Universiteit, Amsterdam. *Renal Unit, Academical Medical Center, Amsterdam, The Netherlands.

The aim of this study was to assess the antigen presenting capacity of human peritoneal cells (PC) and especially the role of dendritic cells (DC) versus macrophages (Mϕ). Overnight dialysis fluid of patients undergoing continous ambulatory peritoneal dialysis (CAPD) and peritoneal fluid of healthy women undergoing laparoscopic sterilization were used as sources of PC. PC were cultured for 16h whereafter nonadherent PC (NAC) were separated from adherent PC (Mϕ enriched). Fc-receptor positive cells were removed from the NAC and the remaining cells seperated in a high density (T- and B cell enriched) and low density fraction (DC enriched). The different cellfractions were immunophenotyped and tested for their capacity to present allo-antigen, Candida Albicans extract (CA) and purified protein derivative (PPD).
Results show that 5% (median, range 1-16) of the PC were DC (with no difference between laparoscopy and CAPD material) and that DC could be enriched up to 28 % (median, range 14-44). DC were CD14 negative cells but showed a typical spot-like staining pattern with anti-CD68 whereas Mϕ showed a strong pancytoplasmatic staining pattern. Functionally DC showed a superior antigen presenting capacity for both allo-antigen and CA/PPD as compared to autologous monocytes, CAPD Mϕ and laparoscopy Mϕ. A major difference between CAPD Mϕ and laparoscopy Mϕ was the far better presentation of allo-antigen by CAPD Mϕ. The level of integrines or MHCII as measured semi-quantative on the FACS could not account for this phenomenon. The supernatant of cultured CAPD peritoneal Mϕ did not change the APC activity of DC. When CAPD Mϕ an DC were co-cultured in a double chamber system an enhanced APC activity of low numbers of DC was observed. However this was only part of the respons that was observed when direct cellular contact was possible between CAPD Mϕ and allogeneic T cells.
In conclusion, human PC have a potent antigen presenting capacity due to a relative high percentage of DC. In addition CAPD Mϕ have an increased allo-antigen presenting capacity that is in part mediated by direct cellular contact.

AUTOANTIBODIES TO MACROPHAGE HORMONES (CYTOKINES) DETECTION AND BIOLOGICAL SIGNIFICANCE.

Bendtzen K., Hansen M.B., Diamant M, Svenson M.
Departments of Medicine TTA and Infectious Diseases M, Rigshospitalet University Hospital, Tagensvej 20, DK-2200 Copenhagen N, Denmark.

The presence of specific antibodies to IL-1α and IL-6 in sera of 15 - 75% of normal individuals and in patients with immunoinflammatory disorders has been demonstrated recently. The frequencies of occurrence and their levels are highly variable, suggesting that these antibodies may be involved in physiological and pathophysiological processes. The Fab fragments of the respective antibodies bind IL-1α and IL-6 with exquisite specificity and with remarkably high affinities (Kd: 10^{-11} to 10^{-10} M). The autoantibodies inhibit receptor binding and thus the bioactivities of the cytokines to which they are specifically aimed. They are polyclonally derived, because they are recognized by antibodies to both immunoglobulin light chains. They are almost exclusively of the IgG class, IgG_4 constituting about 50% of the autoantibodies to IL-1α (IgG_4 normally amounts to 1% of total IgG). IgG_4 does not activate complement, and lattice formation is limited with these antibodies. Hence, precipitation of IL-1α/ anti-IL-1α IgG_4 is unlikely to occur to any significant degree *in vivo*. The autoantibodies to IL-1α and IL-6 are the single most important binding proteins of these cytokines in normal human sera.

'Autoantibodies' to other cytokines, e.g. IL-2, TNFα, and the interferons, have been reported in normal individuals. However, it is important to realize that naturally occurring antibodies to cytokines, apart from those against IL-1α and IL-6, not always bind the cytokines in a specific manner or, indeed, with any appreciable affinity. Thus, Western blotting techniques may show some degree of specificity even though the binding between antibody and ligand is weak and topographically unassociated with the specific binding sites of the antibodies.

The biological role of the autoantibodies to IL-1α and IL-6 is not yet understood, although their binding forces suggest that they interfere with immune and inflammatory processes, for example by blocking or destroying antigen-presenting cells carrying membrane-bound cytokine and/or by scavenging bioactive IL-1α and IL-6 released by cells at inflammatory sites. Furthermore, the IgG_4 autoantibodies to IL-1α may function as specific carriers, and thus systemic regulators, of circulating IL-1α. Inappropriate production or function of autoantibodies to inflammatory cytokines may be pathogenetically involved in many inflammatory diseases and, possibly, in systemic complications to infections and trauma. Therapeutic application of these normally occurring antibodies is of obvious clinical interest.

GENETIC ACCESSIBILITY AND ENDOTOXIN RESPONSIVENESS OF THE TNF LOCUS IN MACROPHAGES, FIBROBLASTS, AND HYBRID CELLS

Bruce Beutler, M.D.

In different cell types, a given gene may be active or inactive, as directed by processes that occur during differentiation. As an example, the TNF gene is activated by both lipopolysaccharide and cycloheximide in RAW 264.7 macrophages, whereas neither stimulus activates the gene in 3T3 fibroblasts. This finding would suggest that the TNF gene has been rendered inaccessible to transcription in the 3T3 cell environment. Supporting this conclusion, the methylation pattern of the TNF gene is readily distinguishable in these two cell types: extensive methylation is observed in 3T3 cells, but not in RAW 264.7 cells. Yet inaccessibility alone does not explain the silence of the TNF gene within LPS-treated 3T3 cells; the LPS signaling pathway seems to be defective in these cells as well. To test the integrity of LPS signaling, we used a CAT reporter construct containing the TNF promoter, 5'-UTR, and 3'-UTR. This reporter responds to cycloheximide when permanently transfected into 3T3 cells, suggesting that it remains accessible in this environment; however, it fails to respond to LPS, in both permanent and transient transfection studies. 3T3 cells thus lack essential components of the LPS signaling pathway. When RAW 264.7 cells are fused with 3T3 cells, the hybrid cell population fails to produce TNF in response to LPS. As in the 3T3 parent, the TNF gene becomes highly methylated, no longer responds to induction by LPS, and is only weakly responsive to cycloheximide. Moreover, the endotoxin signaling pathway is largely abrogated, as assessed by transient transfection with LPS-responsive CAT reporter constructs. It would therefore appear that 3T3 cells are able to silence the TNF gene, as well as the LPS signaling pathway, through exercise of a specific, dominant mechanism. The DNA sequences targeted within the TNF gene are apparently not included in the reporter transgene construct, which remains accessible to a far greater extent than the TNF gene itself.

ICAM 1-SURFACE EXPRESSION IS AN EARLY PARAMETER OF MACROPHAGE ACTIVATION IN PULMONARY SARCOIDOSIS

S Bohnet, B Kreft, J Braun, K Dalhoff
Med. University Luebeck, Departments of Internal Medicine and Medical Microbiology

Pulmonary sarcoidosis is characterized by a mononuclear cell alveolitis with granuloma formation. The interaction between alveolar macrophages (AM) and CD4+- lymphocytes, which is crucial in the pathogenesis of this disease, is still incompletely understood.
We investigated the surface expression of ICAM-1 on AM using a sandwich ELISA technique in comparison to immunocytochemical staining. Cells were isolated from 10 patients with sarcoidosis (type 1: n=7, type 2: n=3) undergoing bronchoalveolar lavage and from 6 healthy volunteers. Furthermore, parameters of macrophage activation and lymphocyte recruitment (TNF-bioassay, lymphocyte percentage and CD4-count in the lavage) were measured as well.
Patients with sarcoidosis showed significantly increased ICAM-1 surface expression as compared to the controls (0.74 EU ± 0.27 vs 0.46 EU ± 0.12, $p < 0.01$). The results were confirmed by immunoalkaline staining (78% ±11 vs 40% ± 8 positive cells).
ICAM-1 expression on AM from patients with sarcoidosis correlated with the spontaneous release of TNF ($r = 0.77$, $p < 0.05$), whereas no relationship to lymphocyte percentage or CD4 - count in the lavage was observed.
,In summary, the increased ICAM-1 expression on AM, which could be demonstrated even in early stages of the disease, is correlated rather to the state of macrophage activation than to the lymphocytic part of the alveolitis.

IMMUNOMODULATING PROPERTIES OF A ROYAL JELLY ACID, THE HYDROXY-10, DECEN-2, TRANSOIC ACID (DHA) AND OF DHA-GLYCEROL DERIVATIVES, ON A MACROPHAGE CELL LINE

C. BOTTEX-GAUTHIER(1), F. PICOT(2), M. BENECHIE(2), D. VIDAL(1) and P. POTIER(2)

(1) CRSSA, Unité de Microbiologie, 38702 LA TRONCHE CEDEX, FRANCE.
(2) CNRS-ICSN, 91198 GIF-SUR-YVETTE CEDEX, FRANCE.

Macrophage can be triggered by susbtances which potentiate the specific as well the non specific immunity. This activation is modulated by a cascade of events, involving the induction of cytokine secretion, such as TNF-α, and the production of reactive oxygen intermediates. In the present study, we investigated the immunomodulating properties of a fatty acid, one of the major components of royal jelly, the hydroxy-10, decen-2, transoic acid (DHA), on a macrophage cell line. Several parameters were studied : the dehydrogenase mitochondrial activity, DNA synthesis, TNF-α secretion and H_2O_2 production. Concurrently with royal jelly, we investigated the effects of DHA-glycerol derivatives in J774.1 cells. A mono-DHA glycerol, a di and a tri-DHA glycerol were assayed in concentrations ranging from 100 µg/ml to 0.012 µg/ml. DHA and mono DHA-glycerol derivative induced a significant stimulation of mitochontrial metabolism of J774.1 cells for all concentrations assayed. Di and tri-DHA glycerol derivatives exerted a strong cytotoxic effect for concentrations above 25 µg/ml. Royal jelly did not trigger any stimulation of mitochondrial metabolism in the same dose range. In addition, DHA-glycerol derivatives effectively stimulated DNA synthesis in J774.1 cells, whereas royal jelly and DHA did not. We observed a significant TNF-α production when J774.1 cells were stimulated with DHA-glycerol derivatives though DHA alone induced TNF-α secretion, but to a lesser extent. Finally, preliminary results concerning H_2O_2 secretion, upon stimulation with DHA or DHA-Glycerol derivatives are presented. These data suggest that coupling the active component to a lipophilic vehicle (glycerol) may potentiate the transmembrane pathway of the drug and improve its immunomodulating properties.

The role of microglia cells in viral infections

R. Brinkmann, J. Sedgwick, S. Schwender, H. Imrich, R. Dörries and V. ter Meulen
Institut für Virologie und Immunbiologie, Universität Würzburg, Versbacher Str. 7, D - 8700 Würzburg, Germany

The control of viral infections of the central nervous system (CNS) is dependent on an effective immune surveillance. In this context microglia cells may play a major role since these cells are closely related to peripheral macrophages. However, despite their possible importance in immune reactions in the CNS only little information is available about these cells due to the lack of proper isolation procedures. Recently, we have developed a method to isolate microglia cells from neonatal and adult brain which allows us to characterize these cells in relation to viral infections. We started to investigate microglia cells in rats infected with coronavirus as well as in rhesus monkey and in man infected with simian immunodeficiency virus (SIV) or human immunodeficiency virus (HIV), respectively. In rats, residing microglia cells respond to inflammation by proliferation and upregulation of CD45, CD4 and MHC class I molecules. In SIV and HIV infection, microglia is latently infected, but the infection turns productive after prolonged tissue culture passages. No major differences between microglia and macrophages were seen by evaluating the phenotype of these cells on the basis of cell surface markers. However, cytokine synthesis is different in microglia and macrophages with and without virus infection. These findings support the hypothesis that microglia, although derived from bone marrow precursor cells have differentiated in the CNS into a cell population which is different from peripheral macrophages. Moreover, the data obtained on cytokine synthesis of microglia after SIV/HIV infection indicate that cytokines are primed candidates as mediators of some of the adverse effects seen in Neuro-AIDS.

MYELIN P2 PROTEIN INDUCES PROINFLAMMATORY CYTOKINES mRNA ACCUMULATION AND SECRETION BY HUMAN CULTURED PHAGOCYTES.

Pierluigi BARON*, Gabriela CONSTANTIN* and Marco A. CASSATELLA §
*Institute of Neurology, University of MILANO, and §Institute of General Pathology, University of VERONA, ITALY.

P2 is a basic protein which is found in peripheral nervous system (PNS) myelin. P2 is known to produce the induction of experimental allergic neuritis (EAN). EAN is an inflammatory demyelinating polyneuropathy that, for its similar clinical features and inflammatory lesions, represents a close animal model of acute human Guillain-Barre' syndrome. Since macrophages are the predominant inflammatory cell type present in the PNS during EAN, we wanted to find out whether mononuclear phagocytes were able to generate proinflammatory mediators upon interaction with P2. For this purpose we treated human cultured monocytes or monocyte-derived macrophages (MDM) with purified bovine P2 protein, and, to make a comparison, with LPS. Northern blot analysis and specific ELISAs demonstrated that the P2 protein induced a time dependent mRNA accumulation and secretion of Tumor Necrosis Factor (TNF) and Interleukin-8 (IL-8). Cytokine production was also obtained with a purified rabbit P2 protein, and was not influenced by polymixin B, which, on the other hand, in parallel experiments, almost completely abolished the action of LPS. In addition, P2 protein was found unable to trigger the release of H_2O_2 by monocytes or by MDM, even though phagocytes had been previously activated by an exposure to IFN-γ for 24-48 h, before P2 stimulation. Our results could suggest that the release of proinflammatory cytokines by human phagocytes, upon stimulation with P2 protein, may have an important role in the effector mechanisms underlying demyelination during EAN.

CORRELATION BETWEEN INTRACELLULAR CALCIUM ELEVATION AND O_2^- RELEASE IN RESPONSE TO F-MET-LEU-PHE IN U-937 AND HL-60 CELLS.

Jean-Luc BUEB and Eric J. TSCHIRHART. Neuroimmunologie & Inflammation, Centre de Recherche Public - Santé. 120, route d'Arlon. L-1150 LUXEMBOURG.

Phagocytes possess an enzymatic complex, the NADPH oxidase, which is able to catalyse the one-electron reduction of molecular oxygen to superoxide O_2^-, the initial product of the respiratory burst. O_2^- release can be induced by f-Met-Leu-Phe (fMLP) in neutrophil-like cells HL-60, and in macrophage-like cells U-937. The purpose of this work was to study the mobilization of intracellular calcium in parallel with O_2^- release in these cells following induction of the respiratory burst by fMLP or phorbol myristate acetate (PMA).

HL-60 and U-937 cells were grown in Iscove's and RPMI-1640 medium supplemented with 15% FCS and 5% newborn calf serum (NCS), and 5% FCS and 5% NCS, respectively. Cell differentiation was induced by dimethyl-sulfoxide (DMSO, 1.3%) for 4 days (HL-60) or 2 days (U-937). Using this method, HL-60 differentiate into neutrophil-like cells and U-937 into macrophage-like cells. O_2^- release was measured after one hour using the ferricytochrome *c* reduction method. Intracellular calcium variations were monitored using Fura-2, after loading the cells (2×10^6) with the acetoxy-methyl-ester of Fura-2 at 2.5 μM for 30 minutes. fMLP (10^{-7} M) induced O_2^- release in differentiated but not in resting U-937 cells (0.62 ± 0.13 nmoles O_2^- /10^6 cells compared to 0.04 ± 0.02 nmoles O_2^- /10^6 cells). fMLP (10^{-5}M) induced a rise in intracellular calcium from 44-46 nM to 325-331 nM in differentiated cells compared to 120-169 nM to 500-578 nM in resting ones. PMA (10^{-7}M) induced O_2^- release in DMSO-differentiated U-937 cells but not in resting cells (2.08 ± 0.32 nmoles O_2^- /10^6 cells compared to 0.10 ± 0.10 mm O_2^- /10^6cells), whereas there was no difference in intracellular calcium variations between resting and DMSO-differentiated cells following PMA stimulation. fMLP (10^{-7}M) induced a higher respiratory burst in differentiated than in resting HL-60 cells (0.69 ± 0.25 nmoles O_2^- /10^6 cells compared to 0.43 ± 0.28 nmoles O_2^- /10^6 cells). fMLP (10^{-5}M) induced an important rise in intracellular calcium from 75-98 nM to 1135-1265 nM in differentiated cells compared to 45-57 nM to 197-371 nM in resting ones. PMA (10^{-7}M) induced O_2^- release in quiescent cells and in DMSO-differentiated cells (5.32 ± 1.40 nmoles O_2^- /10^6 cells compared to 6.19 ± 1.41 nmoles O_2^- /10^6 cells respectively). PMA (10^{-7}M)-induced calcium modifications were similar in resting and in differentiated HL-60 cells.

These results indicate that differentiation of U-937 and HL-60 cells promotes a more efficient coupling of the fMLP receptor with the NADPH oxidase system. This more efficient coupling is linked to a profound increase in intracellular calcium concentration following addition of fMLP, effects which are both more pronounced in HL-60 than in U-937 cells.

EFFECT OF PROTEIN KINASE INHIBITORS ON TANNIN-MEDIATED ARACHIDONIC ACID RELEASE FROM RABBIT ALVEOLAR MACROPHAGES.

Benôit Desrues and Michael S. Rohrbach, Thoracic Diseases Research Unit, Mayo Clinic/Foundation, Rochester, MN, USA

Recent studies from our laboratory have demonstrated that the condensed tannin present in the occupational air pollutant, cotton mill dust, is a potent agonists for the release of arachidonic acid ($C_{20:4}$) from alveolar macrophages (AMØ), and that it induces $C_{20:4}$ release, in part, by inhibiting the reacylation of free $C_{20:4}$ back into the membrane phospholipids (*Am J Respir Cell Mol Biol* in press, 1992). Other studies from our laboratory have shown that exposure to tannin results in the phosphorylation of at least 9 AMØ proteins, 7 of which are also phosphorylated in response to the protein kinase C activator, PMA (*Mol Cell Biochem* 86:163, 1989). Together these data suggested that tannin-mediated release of $C_{20:4}$ from AMØ may involve activation of protein kinases. To test this hypothesis, the effect of two protein kinase inhibitors, H-7 and staurosporine, on tannin-mediated $C_{20:4}$ release was examined. Pretreatment of the AMØ with H-7 resulted in the dose-dependent inhibition of the subsequent ability of tannin to evoke the release of $C_{20:4}$. The EC_{50} for this inhibition was 35 μM. A maximal inhibition of 55% was observed at 100 μM H-7, the highest concentration tested. Pretreatment of the AMØ with staurosporine also resulted in the dose-dependent inhibition of tannin-mediated $C_{20:4}$ release. The EC_{50} for staurosporine inhibition was 690 nM and a maximal inhibition of 65% was observed at 1 μM staurosporine, the highest concentration tested. Dose-response curves for the tannin-mediated release of $C_{20:4}$ performed in the presence or absence of 1 μM staurosporine indicated that percent inhibition of $C_{20:4}$ in the presence of staurosporine was uniform over the entire tannin dose range. Finally, because exposure to tannin resulted in the loss of the ability of the AMØ to reacylate $C_{20:4}$, the effect of staurosporine on reacylation in tannin-treated cells was examined. These studies revealed that staurosporine-dependent inhibition of tannin-mediated $C_{20:4}$ release was paralleled by a restoration of reacylating activity. In conclusion, these data suggest that the mechanism by which tannin promotes the release of $C_{20:4}$ from AMØ involves the action of a protein kinase and that the action of this kinase is involved the inhibition of the ability of the tannin-exposed cells to reacylate $C_{20:4}$ into the membrane lipids. Although these studies do not directly identify the protein kinase invovled in mediation of $C_{20:4}$ release, protein kinase C is a likely candidate based on the similarities in the previously observed pattern of proteins phosphorylated by tannin and the protein kinase C activator, PMA.

PRIMING AND REGULATION OF THE SYNTHESIS AND FORMATION OF CYTOTOXIC MEDIATORS IN LIVER MACROPHAGES

P. Dieter, P. Ambs, U. Arlt, J. Duyster, E. Fitzke and H. Schwende
Institut für Molekulare Zellbiologie, Mooswaldallee 1-9, 7800 Freiburg, Germany

Macrophages are known to release a wide array of biologically active mediators such as cytokines, eicosanoids, superoxide and nitric oxide. In liver macrophages it has been shown that the formation of cytokines, eicosanoids and nitric oxide can be induced e.g. by LPS while the generation of superoxide and eicosanoids is triggered e.g. by zymosan or phorbol ester. PKC is an essential component in the intracellular signal transduction pathway leading to the formation of some of these mediators. Here we describe the priming and direct effects of LPS, serum and γ-IFN on the synthesis of these mediators.

- Macrophages cultured in the absence of serum are less active to phagocytose zymosan particles and to release eicosanoids and superoxide while their capacity to release inositol phosphates is comparable to macrophages cultured in the presence of serum.
- Addition of LPS to serum-free cultured macrophages had no effect on the phagocytic activity and did not influence the formation of inositol phosphates and PGE_2 but primed macrophages for an enhanced superoxide formation.
- Addition of LPS to macrophages cultured in the presence of serum had no effect on the phagocytic activity; the formation of inositol phosphates and superoxide was slightly enhanced; however, LPS led to a 2-5 fold increase in the release of PGE_2.
- The effect of LPS and other compounds (e.g. TNF-α, γ-IFN) on the release of eicosanoids, superoxide, nitric oxide and TNF-α is under investigation. Additionally, the expression of intracellular components involved in the different signal pathways (e.g. PKC, NADPH oxidase) will be studied.

ADOPTIVE IMMUNOTHERAPY OF WALKER-256 CARCINOSARCOMA WITH ACTIVATED MACROPHAGES BY C.PARVUM, INTERFERON AND PHOTO-DYNAMIC THERAPY .

V.F.Dima[1], V.Vasiliu[2], D.Laky[3], P.Ionescu[4]
Cantacuzino-Institute (1), Institute of Atomic Physics (2)
Victor Babes Institute (3), Central Military Hospital (4)
Bucharest - Romania .

The paper aimed at studying the antitumor effects of in vitro interferon activated macrophages (Mu rIFN-gamma-AMØ) or in vivo with C.parvum activated macrophages (C.parvum-AMØ) as compared to macrophages prelevated from rats with Walker-256 tumours, 12 days after transplant and activated by photodynamic therapy (PDT-AMØ) .

The activation degree of macrophages was evaluated by means of the four experimental parameters. We used 4 batches of animals with Walker-256 carcino-sarcoma. Control and treated animals were studied 45 days after transplant.

The obtained results revealed the following : a) macrophages activated with 3 immunopotentiators (C.parvum, IFN-gamma and PDT) had a strong bio-logical activity (phagocytary, metabolic and cytotoxic) ; b) they inhibited tumor evolution ; c) an increased survival rate, e.g. 78.3% in the batch treated with C.parvum-AMØ ; 70.6% in IFN-AMØ as compared to 65.9% survival rate in animals within the batch treated with PDT-AMØ and in contrast with the survival rate of rats within the untreated (control-batch) Walker-256 tumours, which was 13.9% .

Adoptive immunotherapy with C.parvum, IFN and PDT activated macrophages induced tumor regression in 11± 3.5 days and their disappearance after 22± 5.3 days since the beginning of the treatment.

Conclusions : in animals treated with adoptive immunotherapy the following were noticed : a) an increased biological activity of macrophages ac-tivated with the 3 immunopotentiators (C.parvum, IFN and PDT); b) an increased survival rate and c) a significant antitumor activity varying from a reduction of tumor volume to complete recovery .

Being simple, safe and lacking side effects active immunotherapy with photobioactivated macrophages might be extensively used in oncologic clinics for cancer treatment .

MEMBRANE ASSOCIATED C-REACTIVE PROTEIN EXPRESSION BY MACROPHAGES

Christine Egenhofer, Karin Fehsel and Victoria Kolb-Bachofen

Institute for Immunobiology, Fac. of Medicine, Heinrich-Heine-University, DÜSSELDORF, Germany.

C-reactive protein (CRP) is an acute phase marker belonging to the pentraxin family. During infections or inflammations serum concentrations raise rapidly and early in man and to a lesser degree also in rats.

We could show, that CRP occurs as a membrane-associated protein (mCRP) constitutively expressed on rat liver macrophages (Kupffer cells), representing the galactose-specific receptor activity on the surface of rat liver macrophages. This receptor mediates effectively the endocytosis of particulate ligands exposing multiple galactosyl groups on their surface.

Monoclonal antibodies, which recognize a neo-epitope on rat CRP present on protein subunits but not on native serum CRP (sCRP) and polyclonal antisera against native sCRP which do not recognize subunits have been used to investigate the mCRP on Kupffer cells: Indirect immunoperoxidase labelling reveals positive staining of Kupffer cells by the monoclonal antibodies against subunits but not by the polyclonals against the native pentamer. The same mCRP expression was found on alveolar macrophages and activated peritoneal macrophages as well as on rat and human monocytes after culture on glass surface.

Rat Kupffer cells synthesize their own mCRP: With RNA-RNA in situ hybridization using a human CRP-clone we obtained positive signals in the macrophages. In addition a positive in situ hybridization signal was also found in cryostat sections of rat liver in both: hepatocytes as well as Kupffer cells. 18 hours after i.v. injection of C. parvum Kupffer cells and hepatocytes showed an enhanced hybridization signal. Extrahepatic synthesis of CRP was found in rat alveolar macrophages and human monocytes.

In conclusion we here describe data which show that rat liver macrophages synthesize and express membrane-associated mCRP with a conformation different from serum CRP (sCRP). The mode of expression suggests, that mCRP can also serve as a marker for inflammatory macrophages.

MODULATION OF INTERCELLULAR ADHESION MOLECULES ON TPA-INDUCED U937 MONOCYTIC CELLS BY GLUCOCORTICOIDS.

Emmendörffer, A.[1], Raeder, E.[1], Hoff, T.[2], Spencker, T.[2], Lohmann-Matthes, M.-L.[1], and Goppelt-Strübe, M.[2]
[1] Fraunhofer Institute Hannover, Dept. of Immunobiology
[2] Medical School Hannover, Dept. of Molecular Pharmacology

The human monocytic cell line U937 served as model system to monitor the effects of glucocorticoids on the monocytic differentiation. Differentiation of U937 cells to morphologically and functionally macrophage-like cells was induced by incubation with the phorbolester TPA. Since incubation with TPA resulted in a monolayer of adherent, non-proliferating U937 cells, we investigated by flow cytometry whether the expression of cell surface receptors like intercellular adhesion molecule-1 (ICAM-1) and the common subunit (ß-chain; CD 18) of LFA-1, Mac-1 and gp150/95 (CD 11c) was changed concomittantly. The results show that during the differentiation process both molecules were upregulated. Preincubation of U937 cells with either dexamethasone (10^{-7}M and 10^{-6}M) or with prednisolone (10^{-7}M and 10^{-6}M) interfered with the TPA-induced phenotypic alterations as monitored by morphology and flow cytometric analysis. The cells kept their rounded structure and the expression of ICAM-1 and CD 18 was reduced. Incubation with progesterone, however, did not influence the TPA-induced phenotypic alterations. Furthermore, incubation of fully differentiated U937 cells with glucocorticoids resulted in a decreased expression of ICAM-1 and CD 18, corresponding to reduced adherence of the cells. In conclusion these data show that besides several other effects glucocorticoids modulate the differentiation of monocytic cells and alter expression of adhesion molecules. This might contribute to the anti-inflammatory and immunosuppressive effects of these compounds.

RM3/1 SURFACE EXPRESSION ON MONOCYTES IS DIRECTLY CORRELATED TO GLUCOCORTICOID RECEPTOR BINDING AFFINITY.

U. Erpenstein, P. Rohdewald*, C. Sorg; Institute of Experimental Dermatology, von-Esmarch-Str.56, and *Pharmaceutical Chemistry, 4400 Münster, FRG

The RM3/1 antigen is expressed on a monocyte/macrophage subpopulation during the downregulatory phase of inflammation[1]. This antigen shows highly increased cellsurface expression in the presence of glucocorticoids *in vitro* and *in vivo* [1,2]. We analyzed the relation between RM3/1 antigen expression and glucocorticoids of different receptor binding affinities. Monocytes, isolated from human buffy coats, were cultured for 16 h with five concentrations each of triamcinolone (relative receptor affinity: 1), prednisolone (12), beclomethasone (76), dexamethasone (100), flunisolide (180), triamcinolone acetonide (361), budesonide (935), beclomethasone monopropionate (1200), and fluticasone-17-propionate (1800), respectively. The antigen cellsurface expression was detected by fluorescence flow cytometry using the monoclonal antibody RM3/1. For all tested steroids, a concentration dependent upregulation of the RM3/1 antigen (max. 85%) was recorded as compared to control cells (40%). We found a significant correlation between a definite increase of RM3/1 positive cells and the relative receptor affinity of the different glucocorticoids, as shown by a Pearson's correlation coifficient of 0,83. We conclude that there is a conjoining mechanism of glucocorticoid receptor binding and RM3/1 antigen surface expression.Thus, the RM3/1 antigen, which evidently implies steroid responsivness of monocytes, is a suitable *in vitro* parameter to investigate different immunmodulating effects of glucocorticoids, especially from a clinical standpoint.

[1]Zwadlo G, Voegeli R, Schulze Osthoff K, Sorg C (1987) Expl Cell Biol 55: 295-304

[2] Zwadlo-Klarwasser G, Bent S, Haubeck HD, Sorg C, Schmutzler W (1990) Int Arch Allergy Appl Immunol 91: 175-180

FUNCTIONAL MORPHOLOGY OF SUBARACHNOIDAL MACROPHAGES IN AN EXPERIMENTAL ACUTE MENINGITIS MODEL

P.M. Faustmann[1], D. Krause[2], R.Dux[1], C.W. Zimmermann[1], R. Dermietzel[2]

[1]Department of Neurology, University of Essen and [2]Institute of Anatomy, University of Regensburg

Polymorphonuclear leukocytes (PMN) and cells of the mononuclear-macrophage lineage (MML) play an essential role in the manifestation of acute meningeal inflammatory response. Cells of the MML secrete endogenous mediators, e.g. cytokines, of the inflammatory reaction in the subarachnoidal space and stimulate PMN extravasation. Subarachnoidal macrophages (SAM) are one subclass of the MML and have receptors for IgG and complement. We studied the role of SAM in an experimental acute meningitis model. Meningitis was induced by subarachnoidal application of the complement-C5a-fragment in rabbits. Within one hour of stimmulation increased numbers of PMN and of cells of the MML were detected in the cerebrospinal fluid (CSF) by flow cytometry. This indicates an acute inflammatory reaction. After intracardial perfusion with a fixative and preparation of the tissue, subarachnoidal spaces and meninges were investigated using transmission electron microscopy. SAM were identified between the collagen and the pial cells. In serial sections SAM and PMN were found in interaction via pseudopodia. In addition SAM could be found close to or inserting pseudopodia into the basal lamina of the marginal glia. No interaction between the SAM and the pial cells were observed within this acute stage of inflammation.

We conclude that in the early stages of acute meningitis intercellular actions of SAM and PMN, as well as SAM and the basal lamina of the marginal glia play an important role in the mediation of the inflammatory response.

CYTOKINE INTERACTIONS IN THE GROWTH OF MYELOID PRECURSOR CELLS

Willem E.Fibbe, J.C.Kluin-Nelemans, J.H.F.Falkenburg and R.Willemze
Lab. of Experimental Hematology, Leiden University Medical Center, The Netherlands

Although the proliferative action of the CSF's on responding target cells is direct and mediated by specific receptors on the cell surface, there are many examples of interactions between different CSF's. Several examples of synergistic or inhibitory interactions between GM-CSF and other cytokines will be discussed.
The indirect synergistic action between IL-1 and GM-CSF. The addition of IL-1 alpha to bone marrow cultures stimulated with GM-CSF results in higher numbers of granulocytic colonies, having no effect on monocytic colony growth. This synergistic activity is not present anymore when CD34-purified bone marrow cell suspensions are used. Neutralization experiments with an anti-IL-6 antiserum showed no effect of the antiserum on granulocytic colony growth. In contrast, the addition of an anti-G-CSF monoclonal antibody completely abrogates the synergy between IL-1 and GM-CSF. These results indicate that the increase in CFU-G growth is due to the synergistic action between GM-CSF and IL-1-induced G-CSF. **The direct inhibitory interaction between IL-4 and GM-CSF.** As a single factor, IL-4 has no colony-stimulating activity. However, on human bone marrow cells stimulated with GM-CSF, addition of IL-4 results in a reduction to 10-20% of the number of CFU-M, while the number of CFU-G colonies is not affected. This effect is preserved in cultures of CD34-purified cells, suggesting a direct effect on progenitor cells. Since IL-4 down regulates the production of IL-6 in monocytes, we tested whether addition of IL-6 could overcome the IL-4 induced inhibition. A partial reversal of inhibition was observed, indicating that down regulated production of IL-6 may contribute to the IL-4 induced inhibition of CFU-M growth. **The permissive role of IL-6 on GM-CSF stimulated CFU-M growth.** Since monocytes are potent producers of IL-6, the role of auto-and paracrine production of IL-6 on the development of colonies was studied. The addition of an anti-IL-6 antibody to cultures of bone marrow cells stimulated with GM-CSF resulted in a 50% reduction in the number of CFU-M, whereas the number of granulocytic colonies was unaffected. This effect was preserved in cultures of CD34-positive bone marrow cells and could be reversed by the addition of excess concentrations of IL-6. Interestingly, the addition of an anti-IL-6-receptor (80 kd chain) blocking monoclonal antibody resulted in an almost complete inhibition of monocytic colony formation. This inhibitory effect could be partiallly overcome by adding excess concentrations of IL-6. Addition of IL-6 was able to enhance monocytic colony formation in serum-deprived cultures. These results show that IL-6 is a permissive factor for monocytic colony growth. **Conclusion:** The different interactions between growth factors in bone marrow cultures illustrate a complex network, where enhancing or inhibiting activities depend on the lineage of the progenitor cell, the type of growth factor used to induce colony formation, and the presence of accessory cells. Many activities of HGF are due to intermediate production of other HGF, that may serve as synergistic, inhibitory or permissive factors.

EFFECTS OF IL-10 ON HUMAN MONOCYTE FUNCTION.

Carl G. Figdor, René de Waal Malefijt*, Anje A. te Velde, Jan E. de Vries*
Division of Immunology, The Netherlands Cancer Institute,
Plesmanlaan 121, 1066 CX Amsterdam, The Netherlands,
and *DNAX Research Institute of Molecular and Cellular Biology,
Palo Alto, CA 94304-1104, U.S.A.

We previously observed that IFNγ and IL-4 have different regulatory effects on two different monocyte mediated functions: antigen presentation, and antibody mediated cellular cytotoxicity (ADCC). This is reflected by the cell surface expression of MHC class II and Fcγ receptors, respectively. IFNγ stimulates expression of these molecules at the cell surface of monocytes whereas IL-4 stimulates MHC class II expression but reduces Fcγ receptor expression. We now observed that also IL-10 dramatically alters monocyte function. We observed that in contrast to IFNγ and IL-4 this cytokine downregulates MHC class II expression, which is associated with diminished antigen presenting capacity. In addition we demonstrated that IL-10 is also produced by human monocytes and that it has an autoregulatory function with respect to the synthesis of other monocyte produced cytokines. Finally we observed that IL-0 stimulates Fcγ receptor-1 expression, which correlates with increased ADCC activity.

Together, these results show that IFNγ, IL-4 and IL-10 have different regulatory effects on the antigen presenting capacity and ADCC activity of human monocytes.

THE NOVEL SUBSET OF CD14+/CD16+ BLOOD MONOCYTES IS EXPANDED IN SEPSIS PATIENTS:

G. Fingerle[1], A. Pforte[2], B. Passlick[3], M. Blumenstein[4], M. Ströbel[1], and H.W.L. Ziegler-Heitbrock[1]. [1]Institute for Immunology, Goethestr. 31, [2]Dep. Internal Medicine, Klinikum Innenstadt, [3]Dep. Surgery, Klinikum Innenstadt [4]Dep Internal Medicine, Klinikum Großhadern. University of Munich, 8000 Munich, Germany

Staining with CD14 and CD16 monoclonal antibodies will identify 2 monocyte subpopulations in human blood: a major population of regular monocytes, which strongly expresses the CD14 antigen and a minor population (42 ± 30 cells/mm³, 9.7 % of all monocytes) with weak expression of CD14 and strong expression of the CD16 antigen. In septicemia patients, these CD14+/CD16+ cells can become a major population with more than 50 % of all monocytes in 3/18 patients and with more than 250 cells in 7/18 cases. The remaining CD14++ regular monocytes showed a substantial decrease in CD14 antigen density in 9/11 patients. Three color immunofluorescence demonstrate that the CD14+/CD16+ monocytes in septicemia patients when compared to the CD14++ monocytes exhibit a higher level of class II antigen and a lower level of CD11b and CD33 antigens, consistent with a more mature nature of the CD14+/CD16+ cells. Levels of interleukin-6 were increased in septicemia patients and 3/4 patients with high numbers of CD14+/CD16+ cells (>250/mm³) had high levels of IL-6 (>300/U/ml). These data suggest that septicemia may lead to substantial changes in blood monocyte composition and this may be related to elevated levels of cytokines like IL-6.

MACROPHAGES AS TARGET AND EFFECTOR CELLS DURING IN VITRO INFECTION BY *TOXOPLASMA GONDII*: THE INTERACTION WITH HELPER T CELLS DETERMINES MACROPHAGE ANTIPARASITIC ACTIVITY

H.G. Fischer, G. Reichmann, B. Nitzgen, K. Dick, W. Däubener and U. Hadding, Inst. für Med. Mikrobiologie und Virologie, Heinrich-Heine-Universität, D 4000 Düsseldorf, FRG.

To analyze intercellular signals which form the immune response in toxoplasmosis a murine in vitro model has been established by co-cultures of macrophages (Mϕ) with T cells and viable parasites. Tachyzoites of the highly virulent *Toxoplasma gondii* strain BK were used at a lethal dose permitting at least one cycle of intracellular multiplication during the assay. As appropriate targets peritoneal exudate Mϕ were preferentially infected and proved to control parasite growth following interaction with T cells. As regulatory elements within this 3-party system *Toxoplasma*-specific CD4+ T cell lines or clones were introduced which had been derived from mice immunized with *Toxoplasma* lysate antigen: 3Tx T line cells recognize in the context of $A_\alpha^b A_\beta^k$ MHC class II molecules a < 31 kD common antigen of tachyzoites from both high- and low-virulent strains which is also contained in brain cysts of infected mice. According to their cytokine pattern, 3Tx cells and a series of clones tested represent typical T_H1 cells secreting high titers of IFNγ and LT/TNF-activity and no IL4 or IL6, whereas two T_H2 clones tested produced much IL4 and IL6 and only minute levels of IFNγ or LT/TNF-activity.
Within the complete infection culture, antigenic T cell activation at the one end of the reaction cascade was monitored by measuring IL3, while the growth of toxoplasms at the other end was evaluated simultaneously via the uptake of tritiated uracil. As an important mechanism of Mϕ toxoplasmostatic effector function the synthesis of nitrogen oxides was demonstrated to cause total growth inhibition and to be induced by the presence of activated T cells. Graded paralysis of this antiparasitic pathway revealed a direct correlation between the burden of infection and the level of Mϕ activation required to overcome it. The crucial role of T cell help was manifested by blocking T cell activation with an anti-Ia mab resulting in uncontrolled increase of toxoplasms. In comparison, co-cultures of infected Mϕ with T_H1 cells showed a reduced parasite growth, whereas those with T_H2 cells failed to influence the progress of in vitro infection. Thereby the presence of TH1 cells could be replaced by the cytokine cocktail produced upon mitogenic stimulation, however none of the individual cytokines proved to provide the full antitoxoplasmic efficacy.
Further studies to elucidate the cytokine-mediated Mϕ activation and to characterize the antiparasitic capacity of Mϕ from different origins are in progress.

Supported by the DFG, project B8, SFB 194

A FIBROSIS INHIBITING THERAPY BY MACROPHAGE STIMULATION IN MYELOFIBROSIS AND LIVERFIBROSIS

Fleischer J, Wolf H, Mohr B, Keck G; Department Haematology/Oncology, Clinic Internal Medicine, Medical Faculty T. University, Dresden, Germany

We demonstrated the antifibrotic and thioacetamide liver cirrhosis-inhibiting effect of clofazimin (Cl) (Ciba-Geigy, Basel). This effect was referred to the stimulation of Kupffercellfunction. Therefore, Zymosan (Z) was applied additionally as macrophage irritant and clearly intensified the clofazimin effect. working hypothesis: on the top of stimulation the Kupffercells produce an inhibitoring factor to leucotrienes or TGF Beta or these cytokines are inhibiting themselves functionally. We determined superoxideanions, leucotriens, PG E2 for characterisation of Kupffercells. The levels of lipidperoxydate, hydroxyproline, N-acetyl-B-D-glucosaminidase, procollagen-III-peptide in liver tissue confirmed the cirrhosis-inhibiting effect of Cl and Z.
We used Cl alone in patients with myelofibrosis. In single cases in cell-rich stage the megakaryocytosis and the cell content were diminished. The erythrocytopoiesis improved in several patients with solitary loss of necessity of blood transfusions. Now examinations of liver biopsy and peripheral blood especially, before and after Interferon: hydroxyproline, pro-collagen-III-peptide, IL 1 and 6, PG E 2, TNF, leucotriens. Comparison with Interferon literature-results.

IDENTIFICATION OF MACROPHAGE ADHESION MOLECULES BY MONOCLONAL ANTIBODY STRATEGY.

Iain Fraser, Derralynn Hughes and Siamon Gordon

Sir William Dunn School of Pathology ; University of Oxford South Parks Road ; Oxford ; OX1 3RE ; UK

Cells of the mononuclear phagocyte system use a range of plasma membrane receptors to interact with both their extracellular environment, as well as with other cells. These receptors are implicated in processes as diverse as constitutive and elicited migration of monocytes from the circulation, endocytosis, signalling, antigen presentation and less well defined trophic interactions with other cells (1). Raising mAb that interfere with these functions provides a strategy for the characterisation of the participating molecules on the macrophage surface. Screening hybridoma supernatants for their ability to inhibit macrophage binding to bacteriologic plastic generated mAb 5C6 (2). In addition to this inhibitory activity in vitro, 5C6 inhibits macrophage and neutrophil recruitment in vivo (3). We have expanded upon this strategy to identify additional, non-integrin molecules involved in macrophage adhesion. mAb 2F8 inhibits the divalent cation-independent adhesion of macrophages to tissue culture plastic surfaces. Ongoing functional and biochemical studies of the 2F8 antigen as a novel macrophage adhesion receptor will be presented.

References

1) S. Gordon et al ; Curr. Opin. Immunol. 4:25-32 (1992)
2) H. Rosen and S. Gordon ; J. Exp. Med. 166:1685-1701 (1987)
3) H. Rosen ; J. Leuk. Biol. 48:465-469 (1990)

THE EFFICIENT BOVINE INSULIN PRESENTATION CAPACITY OF GM-CSF-ACTIVATED BONE MARROW-DERIVED MACROPHAGES CORRELATES WITH A DIMINISHED PROTEASE ACTIVITY AND A HIGH LEVEL OF INTRACELLULAR REDUCING AGENTS

Stefanie Frosch, Ursula Bonifas, Hans-Peter Eck*, W. Droege*, and A.B. Reske-Kunz. Institut für Immunologie, Joh. Gutenberg Universität, Obere Zahlbacher Straße 67, 6500 Mainz. *Abteilung Immunchemie, Deutsches Krebsforschungszentrum, Im Neuenheimer Feld 280, 6900 Heidelberg.

Bone marrow-derived macrophages (BMMph) grown for 10 days in a liquid culture system in the presence of M-CSF can serve as antigen presenting cells capable of stimulating T clone cells and T hybridoma cells with specificity for bovine insulin (BI) to proliferation and/or to IL-2 production. After activation with GM-CSF the macrophages exhibit a drastically higher BI-presentation capacity. Stimulation of BMMph with IFN-τ is less efficient, although these cells express much higher levels of MHC class II molecules compared with GM-CSF-activated BMMph. To investigate whether the different presentation capability of both macrophage populations is based on a different processing capacity we inhibited the activity of several proteases necessary for degradation of the native protein antigen and generation of the antigenic peptide. When serine- and/or thiolproteases were inhibited by chymostatin, leupeptin, or Cbz-Phe-Ala-CHN_2 the BI-presentation potential of IFN-τ-activated BMMph increased drastically and approximated the potential of GM-CSF-stimulated macrophages, while the latter were not influenced by the inhibitors. Upon inhibition of metalloproteases by phosphoramidon BI-presentation function was weakly enhanced in both macrophage populations, while inhibition of acidic proteases with pepstatin A had no influence on BI-presentation. Furthermore, when we pulsed BMMph with BI in the presence of chloroquine or NH_4Cl, substances shown to increase lysosomal pH, IFN-τ-activated macrophages became more efficient presenting cells, while GM-CSF-activated macrophages were not affected. The weaker antigen presenting capacity of IFN-τ-treated BMMph seems to be the consequence of a successive degradation of BI and destruction of antigenic determinants by thiol-/serine proteases. On the other hand, since reduction of disulfide bonds was shown to play a role in the processing of insulin, we measured the levels of the intracellular thiols glutathione and cysteine. BMMph stimulated with GM-CSF have a significantly higher cysteine and glutathione content than IFN-τ-activated BMMph. This high level of thiols and the weak proteolytic cleavage by thiol-/serine proteases may be responsible for the highly efficient BI-presentation capacity of GM-CSF-pulsed BMMph.

PURIFICATION AND CHARACTERIZATION OF MURINE LPS BINDING PROTEIN

P. Gallay, M.P. Glauser, C. Barras, R.J. Ulevitch, P.S. Tobias, J.D. Baumgartner and D. Heumann.

Div. Infectious Diseases, CHUV, Lausanne, Switzerland and Department of Immunology, Scripps Research Institute, La Jolla, CA.

The serum protein, LPS binding protein (LBP), seems to play an important role in regulating host responses to LPS. Complexes of LPS and LBP form in serum and stimulate monocytes/ macrophages or polymorphonuclear leucocytes after binding to CD14. Previous studies have described the structure and properties of LBP from human and rabbit serum. Since mice are used in experimental models of endotoxemia or Gram-negative infections, information is needed about the properties of murine LBP. Murine LBP was purified by ion-exchange and HPLC chromatography and its NH_2-terminal sequence (TNPGLVTRIT) was very similar to human and rabbit LBP (80 to 90% amino acid identity). Murine LBP resembled LBP from other species by promoting the binding of LPS to monocytes and by enhancing the sensitivity of monocytes to LPS at least 100 fold. In mice as in rabbits and humans, LBP was found to be an acute-phase protein. Further studies in vivo in mice using anti-CD14 or anti-LBP reagents will help to understand the role of LBP in response to LPS challenges.

LPS AND CYTOKINE EFFECTS ON TNF-α-mRNA SYNTHESIS IN RAT KUPFFER CELLS

R GAUSLING, M GREWE, HC ESTLER, R HOFFMANN, K GUYFKO and K DECKER
Biochemisches Institut, Hermann-Herder-Straße 7, D-7800 Freiburg, Germany

Kupffer cells (KC) are thought to be the main producers of TNF-α protein within the liver upon stimulation with LPS. This TNF-α release was shown to be inhibited rapidly by PGE_2 and dexamethasone. However, the regulation of TNF-α m-RNA synthesis and the influence of peptide mediators remained undetermined.

Rat liver KC in primary culture were stimulated with LPS (100ng/ml), murine interferon-γ (INF-γ, 50 U/ml), dexamethasone (1μM), PGE_2 (1μM), murine TNF-α (500 U/ml), Il-1ß (100 U/ml), murine Il-6 (150 U/ml) and dBcAMP (1mM) for different periods of time. Total RNA from 1.5-2x 10^6 KC was isolated and Northern blotting was employed using biotinylated riboprobes. Simultaneously, aliquots were reverse-transcribed and semiquantitative PCR was performed (RT-PCR). The identity of the RT-PCR product was established once by Southern blotting.

KC stimulated with LPS/INF-γ showed an appearance for TNF-α-mRNA after 30 min with a maximum between 1h and 2h both in Northern blotting and RT-PCR; after 7h the signal had vanished. Interestingly, the early occurring RNA was 50-100 bases longer than the one detectable at a later stage (approx. 1.44kb). Northern blot analysis of PGE_2-treated KC and also dBcAMP, a stable derivative of the intracellular second messenger of PGE_2, showed a striking inhibition of TNF-α-mRNA synthesis. In contrast, KC treated with LPS + dexamethasone showed hardly a 50% inhibition of TNF-α-mRNA synthesis, although supernatants of cultured cells did not contain significant cytotoxic activity. Moreover, TNF-α itself was able to inhibit LPS-induced TNF-α-mRNA synthesis at a narrow time scale. Even a 24h pretreatment of KC with LPS inhibited an additional endotoxin-evoked TNF-α-mRNA synthesis. Additionally, neither Il-1ß, Il-6 nor INF-γ alone had any effect, but a 24h pretreatment with INF-γ prior to the 90min LPS challenge seemed to have a priming effect for TNF-α-mRNA synthesis. Reverse transcription of mRNA aliquots followed by semiquantitative PCR gave in corresponding results for the various stimuli, thus supporting the data in both mRNA detection assays.

The presented stimulation and suppression experiments demonstrate a regulation of TNF-α production by KC at the mRNA level. The time course of TNF-α-mRNA signals and the inhibition experiments are in full agreement with the data on the release of mature TNF-α obtained with cultured KC. In contrast to other myeloic cells, TNF-α itself was able to inhibit its own TNF-α-mRNA synthesis, while other cytokines did not seem to have an effect. Nevertheless, the detection of TNF-α-mRNA by RT-PCR even in unstimulated KC, the incomplete inhibition of mRNA expression by dexamethasone and the change of the length of mRNA revealed by Northern blot analysis suggest different regulatory mechanisms within the fine-tuning of TNF-α in resting and stimulated KC, respectively.

INHIBITORY EFFECT OF IRON OVERLOAD ON THE BACTERICIDAL ACTIVITY OF MURINE MACROPHAGES IN VITRO

GAUTHIER Y., and ISOARD P.

Unité de Microbiologie - Centre de Recherches du Service de Santé des Armées - B.P. 87 - 38702 LA TRONCHE Cedex - France

The cultivation of resident peritoneal murine macrophages in a medium containing various sources of iron such as human iron-saturated transferrin or lactoferrin, or ammonium ferric citrate leads to a decreased phagocytosis-associated bactericidal activity of theses macrophages against an enteropathogenic strain of E. coli. Iron chelators Deferoxamine and human apo-Transferrin have a similar effect. Identically, the extracellular bactericidal power of PMA activated macrophages is also decreased in the same conditions. These results suggest that the observed inhibitory effect of iron overload is to hinder the expression of some bactericidal mechanisms, rather than increase the formation of free radicals toxic to the cells. Superoxide anion generation and nitrite production are measured under different culture conditions of macrophages.

STIMULATION OF MONOCYTES WITH *MYCOBACTERIUM TUBERCULOSIS*: MODULATION OF SURFACE ANTIGEN EXPRESSION AND INDUCTION OF CELL-ASSOCIATED IL-1β.

Jens GERCKEN, Hans-Dieter Flad, and Martin ERNST. Forschungsinstitut Borstel, Institut für Experimentelle Biologie und Medizin, Parkallee 22, 2061 Borstel, Germany

By means of flow-cytometry analysis we investigated the modulation of monocyte surface molecules as well as the cell-associated production of IL-1β following stimulation with *M.tuberculosis*. Human monocytes were isolated from PBMC by counterflow elutriation, subsequently stimulated with live FITC-labelled *M.tuberculosis* (H37Rv) and cultured for 18h. In order to analyze the expression of surface molecules of cells that have phagocytosed labelled bacteria monocytes were stained with phycoerythrin-labelled monoclonal antibodies. The expression of cell-associated IL-1β was detected by intracellular staining with the IL-1β-specific monoclonal antibody FIB-3 after permeabilization of the cell membrane with n-octyl-β-D-glycopyranoside.

With regard to the modulation of surface molecules we found that the expression of complement receptor 1 (CD35) and of the high affinity Fc_γ-receptor (CD64) is down-regulated on most mycobacteria-infected monocytes. Other surface antigens constitutively present on monocytes, like HLA-DR, CD14, ICAM-1 (CD54), and the β2-integrins (CD11a/b/c) were expressed in similar amounts on phagocytically active and inactive monocytes of the mycobacteria-exposed cultures. In comparison to unstimulated control monocyte cultures, however, antigen densities of CD14, CD54, and CD11c were upregulated.

Intracellular staining with monoclonal antibody FIB-3 revealed that IL-1β is produced by both, phagocytically active and inactive monocytes. A variable amount of the *M.tuberculosis*-infected cells appeared immunofluorescence-negative for IL-1ß. Monocytes having ingested high numbers of bacteria were predominantly immunofluorescence-negative for IL-1β.

Taken together, our results demonstrate that the modulation of surface molecule expression and induction of IL-1β is not restricted to monocytes loaded with mycobacteria. This finding suggests that *M.tuberculosis*-infected monocytes induce phenotypic changes and IL-1β-production in bystander monocytes either by soluble mediators and/or direct cell to cell contact.

This work was supported by BMFT, grant no. 01KI 8827

PRODUCTION OF A NOVEL SOLUBLE MEDIATOR DURING THE INTERACTION OF T_h1-LYMPHOCYTES AND BONE MARROW-DERIVED MACROPHAGES CULTURED IN GM-CSF

T. Germann, E. Rüde,
Institut für Immunologie der Joh. Gutenberg Universität, W-6500 Mainz.

The recognition of MHC molecules in combination with processed fragments of an antigen by the T cell receptor is responsible for the specificity of an immune response and results in partial activation of specific T cells. In addition, accessory signals play an important role in the activation process of T cells. They enhance and modify the T cell receptor signal leading to a stronger and sustained stimulation. Accessory signals can be delivered to T cells either by direct cell contact or by soluble mediators. Macrophages derived from bone marrow cells by culture in GM-CSF-containing medium are very potent antigen-presenting cells for T_h1-lymphocytes, although they express only few MHC class II molecules on their surface. We could demonstrate that these macrophages express an as yet undefined membrane molecule(s) required for the proliferation of T_h1-lymphocytes stimulated via their T cell receptor/CD3-complex. Such an interaction between membrane-bound molecules is also required for the synthesis of a novel soluble mediator during the macrophage-T_h1-lymphocyte interaction. This mediator by itself can then act on T_h1-lymphocytes, further augmenting their activation. Its effects on T_h1-lymphocytes include growth enhancement, stimulation of IFN-τ-synthesis as well as triggering of LFA-1/ICAM-1-dependent cell adhesion. The molecular weight of this factor - about 65 KD on SDS-PAGE - and some other biochemical and functional properties indicate that it is probably identical with the recently described cytokine IL-12. So far we were unable to detect this mediator in supernatants of T_h1-lymphocytes or macrophages stimulated separately by various agents. Furthermore, only GM-CSF seems to induce a functional state in bone marrow-derived macrophages which allows its synthesis upon coculture with T_h1-lymphocytes. Macrophages derived from bone marrow cells cultured in M-CSF (CSF-1) do not possess this functional capacity. However, short-term treatment (24 h) with GM-CSF but not IFN-τ is sufficient to convert them into a functional state allowing the generation of this novel soluble mediator.

ALPHA-METHYLPREDNISOLONE CAN MODULATE LECTINOPHAGOCYTOSIS OF YEASTS BY HUMAN AND MURINE MACROPHAGES.

Jean GIAIMIS[1], Yves LOMBARD[1], Paul FONTENEAU[1], Rachel LEVY[1], Madeleine MAKAYA-KUMBA[1], Philippe POINDRON[1] and Janis LAZDINS[2].
[1]Université Louis Pasteur, Département d'Immunologie, Immunopharmacologie et Pathologie, BP 24, F 67401, ILLKIRCH Cedex, France and [2]Ciba Geigy Limited, Research Department, K125 2.17, CH 4002, BASEL, Switzerland.

Non-opsonized *Saccharomyces cerevisiae* can be phagocytozed by macrophages (human or murine). In the case of mouse peritoneal macrophages, it is believed that this phenomenon is mediated by a β-glucan receptor. Similar results have been obtained using fresh human blood monocytes. However, using *in vitro* differentiated cells, it has been claimed that the phenomenon is mediated by mannose receptors.

Since corticosteroids are known to modulate expression of mannose et β-glucan receptors on murine phagocytic cells, we examined the effect of this substance on human cells. The study was designated as comparative study with murine macrophages.

Freshly isolated and *in vitro* cultured human blood monocytes obtained by combination of leukapheresis and centrifugal elutriation and resident mouse peritoneal macrophages (BALB/c mice) *in vitro* cultured were used for this study.

Lectinophagocytosis was evaluated using methods previously described (Giaimis *et al.*, J. Immunol. Methods, in press, and this conference).

Circulating human monocytes do not express the mannose receptor, therefore, non-opsonic phagocytosis is mediated by β-glucan receptors. When these cells are induced *in vitro* to differentiate, they express the mannose receptor. Culture (7 days) in the presence of α-methylprednisolone (10^{-6}M) induced phagocytosis of much higher amounts of non-opsonized yeast particles than non treated cells. This process could be totally inhibited when during phagocytosis α-mannan and laminarine (400µg/ml) were present, single substances only partly inhibited this process. Therefore, under these conditions, the lectinophagocytosis was mainly mediated by mannose receptors which are increased, whereas that mediated by β-glucan receptors was diminished.

Freshly isolated murine peritoneal macrophages expressed both mannose and β-glucan receptors. After 4-day culture in the presence of corticosteroids, lectinophagocytosis was significantly reduced. This reduction was due to an effect on β-glucan receptor mediated phagocytosis. The mannose receptor mediated phagocytosis was not affected.

Thus, our studies have demonstrated that in human as well as in murine cells, both types of receptors (i.e. mannose and β-glucan) are involved in the phagocytic process and that corticosteroids affect the functionnal expression of these receptors.

BOTH MANNOSE AND β-GLUCAN RECEPTORS ARE INVOLVED IN PHAGOCYTOSIS OF YEASTS BY MURINE MACROPHAGES.

Jean GIAIMIS[1], Yves LOMBARD[1], Paul FONTENEAU[1], Christian MULLER[1], Rachel LEVY[1], Madeleine MAKAYA-KUMBA[1], Janis LAZDINS[2] and Philippe POINDRON[1].
[1]Université Louis Pasteur, Département d'Immunologie, Immunopharmacologie et Pathologie, BP 24, F 67401, ILLKIRCH Cedex, France and [2]Ciba Geigy Limited, Research Department, K125 2.17, CH 4002, BASEL, Switzerland.

Macrophages are known for their capacity to bind and to ingest opsonized particles (opsonophagocytosis). They are also able to bind and to internalize non-opsonized particles (especially microorganisms such as bacteria or yeasts) bearing polyosidic structures on their surface, through endogenous lectin-like receptors (lectinophagocytosis). Two of these lectins are mainly involved : the mannose receptor and the β-glucan receptor. The mannose receptors are trypsin-sensitive and calcium-dependent. In a previous paper (Giaimis *et al.*, J. Immunol. Methods, in press, 1992) we have shown that autoclaved *Saccharomyces cerevisiae* can be used to study both attachment and internalization steps of lectinophagocytosis. Its wall consists essentially of α-mannans and β-glucans. We show here that autoclaved *S. cerevisiae* can be conveniently used to study both mannose receptor- and β-glucan receptor-mediated lectinophagocytosis.

The murine macrophage cell line MALU used for this study was established in our laboratory (Lombard *et al.*, J. Leukocyte Biol., 44, 391-401, 1988). These cells were shown to display mannose receptors on their surface (Muller *et al.*, J. Leukocyte Biol., 43, 165-171, 1988). It was first observed that lectinophagocytosis of *S. cerevisiae* was totally inhibited when MALU cells were pre-incubated in presence of α-mannans (10 mg/ml). Under the same conditions, opsonophagocytosis of *S. cerevisiae* was not impaired. In addition, laminarin, a soluble β-glucan, (10 mg/ml) inhibited by 50 % lectinophagocytosis when used alone. We hypothesized therefore that both receptors were involved in the phenomenon. This was confirmed by the total inhibition of lectinophagocytosis by a mixture of laminarine and α-mannans at a dose of 400 µg/ml each, whereas when used alone, these polysaccharides inhibited only partly the lectinophagocytosis of *S. cerevisiae.* Treating α-mannans by laminarinase, a β-glucanase, resulted in a preparation which now was unable to totally inhibit lectinophagocytosis, indicating that the commercial preparations of α-mannans are contaminated with β-glucans. Treatment of laminarin with α-mannosidase did not modifiy its inhibiting activity.

Both receptors behave quite differently. After being incubated in presence of α-mannans, washed out, and then treated with laminarin, the MALU cells recovered very rapidly their ability to bind and internalize yeasts. After laminarin treatment, washing out, and addition of α-mannans, the MALU cells did not recover the ability to bind and internalize yeasts. Taken together with the results of the kinetic studies of lectinophagocytosis by either receptors, these observations suggested that the mannose receptors recycle whereas the β-glucan receptors cannot. The lectinophagocytosis which was shown to persist after treatment of the cells by trypsin or EGTA was totally abrogated if cells were treated by laminarin before addition of yeasts, and was only marginally affected by α-mannans. This suggested that β-glucan receptors were trypsin-resistant and calcium-independent.

FUNCTIONAL ß-GLYCAN RECEPTOR EXPRESSED BY MICROGLIA IN THE CENTRAL NERVOUS SYSTEM

J. Giaimis*, V. Bocchini §, A. Menghini §, P. Poindron* & C.D. Muller* *

* Département d'Immunologie,Immunopharmacologie et Pathologie & ** Laboratoire de Biophysique U.A. n°491 du CNRS, Université Louis Pasteur, Centre de Recherche Pharmaceutique, ILLKIRCH, FRANCE.
§ Dipartimento di medicina sperimentale e scienze biochimiche
Università Degli Studi di Perugia. Sezione di biologia cellulare e molecolare. PERUGIA, ITALIA.

Microglial cells represent a distinct type of cells in the central nervous system which have phagocytic properties. In the adult, the functions of microglia appear crucial after brain damage when phagocytic cells eliminate cell debris, acting as the scavengers of the brain. In recent years much progress has been made toward a better understanding of the nature and function of microglial cells. Diseases where an active role for microglia has been proposed recently include Alzheimer's disease, the Acquired Immune Deficiency Syndrome(AIDS) and multiple sclerosis. The immune system seems not to be involved in the generation of amyloid plaques in Alzheimer's disease. Yet microglial cells are greatly present in and around amyloid plaques. Does microglia act as an immune network in the CNS?

Only recently has it been possible to obtain pure (>95%) microglial cell cultures and this proved to be a very powerful tool for studying several morphological and functional aspects of these cells and their secretory products. Recently V. Bocchini was able to immortalize murine microglia in a cell line named BV2 [1].

It has been shown in our laboratory that one can easily discriminate between extra- and intracellular phagocytosed yeasts [2]. We here applied the same technology to FACS analysis. BV2 shows high phagocytic power which can be inhibited by free polysugars: slightly by mannan (a poly-mannose) and completely by ß-laminarin (a poly-glucose). This means that BV2 cells express a high level of functional ß-glycan receptors.

1.Blasi E., Barluzzi R., Bocchini V., Mazzolla R. & Bistoni F., (1990), Immortalization of murine microglial cells by v-raf / v-myc carrying retrovirus. *J. Neuroimmunol.*, **27**, 229-237.
2.Giaimis J., Lombard Y., Makaya-Kumba M., Fonteneau P. & Poindron P., (1992), A new simple method for studying the binding and ingestion steps in the phagocytosis of yeast. *J. Immunol. Methods*, in press.

EXPRESSION AND SECRETION OF MACROPHAGE-SPECIFIC PRODUCTS AFTER *IN VITRO* INFECTION OF HUMAN MONOCYTES/MACROPHAGES WITH HIV

W. Glienke[1], H. von Briesen[1], R. Esser[1,2], S. Müller[1], R. Andreesen[2], H. Rübsamen-Waigmann[1]

1) Georg-Speyer-Haus, Paul-Ehrlich-Str. 42-44, 6000 Frankfurt/M. 70 (Germany)
2) Medizinische Klinik I, Hämatologie, Onkologie, Franz-Josef-Strauß-Allee 11, 8400 Regensburg (Germany)

We studied the response of monocytes/macrophages (MO/MAC) to lipopolysaccharide (LPS) or interferon-gamma stimulation with respect to the expression and secretion of macrophage-specific products i.e. macrophage colony-stimulating factor (M-CSF), c-fms, c-sis, tissue factor, TGF-beta, interleukin-6 (IL-6), TNF, interleukin-8 (IL-8) after *in vitro* infection with HIV. A normal expression but decreased secretion of M-CSF was found in HIV-infected MO/MAC compared to uninfected control cells. The expression and secretion of IL-8 was significantly altered in HIV-infected cells. The IL-8 expression was strongly elevated in HIV-infected cells peaking at 4 hours stimulation with LPS. At that time the uninfected control showed only weak expression of IL-8. Other products e. g. tissue factor, c-fms were not modulated after stimulation. These findings may help to understand the role of MO/MAC in the immunological dysfunction seen in HIV-infected patients.

The Georg-Speyer-Haus is supported by the Bundesministerium für Gesundheit and the Hessische Ministerium für Wissenschaft und Kunst.
Supported by the Bundesministerium für Forschung und Technologie.
(BGA III-004-89/FVP 4)

EFFECTS OF GLUCOCORTICOIDS ON THE TPA-INDUCED MONOCYTIC DIFFERENTIATION

M. Goppelt-Struebe*, T. Hoff and T. Spencker, Inst. of Molecular Pharmacology, Medical School Hannover, W-3000 Hannover 61, Germany

The human monocytic cell line U937 was used as a model system to investigate the effects of glucocorticoids on monocytic differentiation. Upon incubation with the phorbol ester TPA for 48 or 72 h, the immature U937 cells ceased to proliferate and became morphologically and functionally macrophage-like. Preincubation of the cells with glucocorticoids (dexamethasone and prednisolone) but not progesterone had marked effects: The cells remained in suspension and developed very little cell-cell interaction. The TPA-induced ability of the cells to release lysozyme or to generate reactive oxygen radicals (determined as reduction of nitroblue tetrazolium) was markedly reduced. The induction of cyclooxygenase activity and thus the ability to release prostanoids was almost completely abolished.

The primary step of TPA induction, the activation and translocation of protein kinase C, however, was not affected by glucocorticoids as determined by activity measurements and Western blot analysis. There was no change in the subsequent TPA-induced induction of the proto-oncogene c-fos. The down-regulation of the differentiation-related proto-oncogenes c-myc and c-myb was the same in cells treated with TPA in the presence or absence of glucocorticoids. Furthermore, no significant effect of glucocorticoids on the TPA-induced growth arrest was observed.

Glucocorticoids thus interfere with TPA-induced functions, which are typical for activated macrophages; however, they do not impair the differentiation process and concomitant growth inhibition of monocytic cells.

This work was supported by grants from the Niedersachsen Stiftung and the Deutsche Krebshilfe
*Present address: University of Erlangen-Nürnberg, Dept. of Medicine IV, Loschgestr. 8 1/2, W-8520 Erlangen, Germany

PHENOTYPIC AND FUNCTIONAL CHARACTERIZATION OF CD64$^-$ MONOCYTES, A MINOR HUMAN MONOCYTE SUBPOPULATION WITH HIGH ANTIGEN-PRESENTING CAPACITY

Evelin GRAGE-GRIEBENOW, Dirk LORENZEN, Hans-Dieter FLAD, and Martin ERNST.

Forschungsinstitut Borstel, Institut für Experimentelle Biologie und Medizin, Parkallee 22, 2061 Borstel, Germany.

The majority (85-95%) of human peripheral blood monocytes expresses the high affinity Fc_γ-receptor (FcR-I, CD64) on their surface while 5-15% lack this antigen.

Monocytes obtained by counterflow elutriation were separated into highly purified CD64$^-$ and CD64$^+$ monocytes by fluorescence-activated cell sorting, using a monoclonal anti-CD64 antibody which does not block the CD64 Fc-receptor function.

The phenotypic analysis of these monocyte subpopulations is summarized in the following table:

	CD64$^-$ monocytes	CD64$^+$ monocytes
size	++	+++
non-specific esterase	++	++
HLA DR	+++	+
CD14	+	+++
latex particle phagocytosis	+	+++

When stimulated with LPS CD64$^-$ monocytes released more IL-1ß but less IL-6 than CD64$^+$ monocytes, whereas stimulation with PPD (purified protein derivative of tuberculin) induced a higher proportion of CD64$^-$ monocytes to produce cell-associated IL-1ß than of CD64$^+$ monocytes (as measured by flow-cytometry using intracellular IL-1ß immunostaining with monoclonal antibody FIB-3). The antigen-presenting capacity of monocyte subpopulations was assessed by PPD pretreatment of isolated monocyte subpopulations and subsequent addition of 300 to 10,000 PPD-primed monocytes to 200,000 autologous CD4$^+$ T-lymphocytes of tuberculin skin test-positive donors. Under these conditions PPD-primed CD64$^-$ monocytes induced more than tenfold the amount of interferon-γ release from T-cells and also a higher proportion of proliferating T-cells than PPD-primed CD64$^+$ monocytes. Our results indicate that CD64$^-$ monocytes, although comprising only a minority of all monocytes, might play an important immunoregulatory role *in vivo* due to their differential monokine-producing capacity and their more efficient accessory functions in antigen-driven T-cell activation.

LPS AND CYTOKINE INDUCED ICAM-1 EXPRESSION OF RAT LIVER MACROPHAGES IS INHIBITED BY PGE$_2$ AND DEXAMETHASONE

GREWE M, BUDNIK A*, BALLHORN A, KRUTMANN J* and DECKER K
Biochemical Institute and *Department of Dermatology, University of Freiburg, Hermann-Herder-Str. 7, 7800 Freiburg

It is known from immunohistological studies that liver sinusoidal cells may express intercellular adhesion molecule-1 (ICAM-1). ICAM-1 plays a pivotal role in direct intercellular communication which is necessary e. g. for antigen presentation by macrophages. Therefore, we investigated regulatory mechanisms involved in ICAM-1 expression by Kupffer cells (KC), the resident liver macrophages.

Rat liver KC were isolated and cultured by pronase/collagenase perfusion followed by centrifugal elutriation. Treatments for 24 h with LPS (100 ng/ml), interferon-γ (IFN-γ, 50 U/ml), TNF-α (500 U/ml), PGE$_2$ (1 μM), PGD$_2$ (10 μM) dexamethasone (1 μM) and neutralizing antibody against TNF-α were carried out with 48 h cultivated KC. At 72 h KC were removed from the culture dishes, incubated with anti-ICAM-1 antibody, FITC-labeled second antibody and were then subjected to FACS analysis. As controls, KC were incubated with mouse IgG$_1$ antibodies instead of anti-ICAM-1 antibodies.

72 h cultivated, unstimulated KC constitutively expressed ICAM-1. A significant upregulation of ICAM-1 expression could be achieved by stimulations with TNF-α = IFN-γ > LPS. Stimulation with LPS plus IFN-γ had an additive effect on this induction. Constitutive ICAM-1 expression was not suppressed by treatment of KC with PGE$_2$ or PGD$_2$, but by dexamethasone. Nevertheless, PGE$_2$ or dexamethasone, but not PGD$_2$ were able to block ICAM-1 induction caused by LPS, TNF-α or IFN-γ. Assuming that TNF-α may be the ICAM-1 inducing mediator after LPS treatment, KC were stimulated with LPS plus neutralizing anti-TNF-α antibody; this treatment resulted in a significantly reduced ICAM-1 induction by LPS.

In conclusion, the presented data clearly indicate that the Kupffer cells of the liver sinusoid express ICAM-1. Induction of ICAM-1 expression after LPS challenge is at least in part mediated by endogenously produced TNF-α, but other LPS-induced second mediators may be involved. IFN-γ which has only weak effects on cytokine and eicosanoid production, serves as a very potent inducer of ICAM-1 expression. ICAM-1 induction could be effectively blocked by glucocorticoids and by PGE$_2$. Interestingly, the effect of PGE$_2$ was not restricted to inhibition of cytokine production after LPS challenge. It may represent a general suppressive mechanism in ICAM-1 regulation.

DETECTION OF TNF-α-mRNA IN SPLENIC DENDRITIC RETICULUM CELLS BY NON-RADIOACTIVE *IN SITU* HYBRIDIZATION

M GREWE, R HOFFMANN, HC ESTLER, K GUYFKO and K DECKER

Biochemisches Institut, Hermann-Herder-Straße 7, D-7800 Freiburg i.Br., Germany

Activated macrophages, monocytes and T-cells are the major sources of the pleiotropic cytokine, TNF-α. Lipopolysaccharides (LPS) are very potent elicitors of TNF-α synthesis. The spleen is thought to participate in the organism's TNF-α production. Splenic macrophages in primary cell culture were shown to express TNF-α-mRNA. However, little is known about the distribution of TNF-α-mRNA-expressing cells *in vivo*. *In situ* hybridization (ISH) is the only technique that enables the morphological demonstration of specific RNA sequences in individual cells in culture or in tissue sections. Therefore, we studied the distribution of TNF-α-mRNA-expressing cells in the LPS-perfused rat spleen by non-radioactive ISH.

Rat spleens were perfused with RPMI medium containing 100 ng LPS/ml for 90 min or with RPMI alone as a negative control. After fixation tissues were routinely processed to paraffin wax. Five μm-thick sections were mounted on 3-aminopropyltriethoxysilan-coated sterile slides. After proteolysis, *in situ* hybridization of TNF-α-mRNA was carried out using digoxigenin-labelled antisense or sense RNA probes generated by *in vitro* transcription. After pretreatment with hybridization buffer alone, hybridization was carried out overnight either with labelled antisense or sense RNA at 42°C using approximately 150 ng probe/μl. After stringency washes, bound probe was detected by alkaline-phosphatase-conjugated anti-digoxigenin antibody. The distribution of cells detected by ISH was compared with the distribution of macrophages identified by immunohistochemistry with monoclonal antibodies against CD 68, rat macrophages and S 100.

With digoxigenin-labelled antisense RNA we were able to obtain a specific signal in individual cells within the splenic white pulp. No signal was detectable in spleens that were perfused with RPMI alone, or hybridized with sense RNA. Comparison with the location of different macrophages within the spleen revealed a similar distribution of dendritic reticulum cells (DRC) detected by S 100 antibody and those cells detected by ISH.

DRC of splenic germinal centers are thought to be involved in the organism's production of TNF-α protein. With our results we have strong evidence that DRC are the primary cells within rat spleen germinal centers to express TNF-α-mRNA upon stimulation with LPS.

A SIMPLE ASSAY FOR THE DETECTION OF LBP ACTIVITIES

U. Grunwald, C. Krüger, J. Schletter, T. Schilling, C. Schütt
Dept. Med. Immunology, Ernst-Moritz-Arndt-University, Greifswald, Germany

CD14 was discovered as a receptor recognizing endotoxin complexed with serum factors. Two proteins are known mediating LPS binding to CD14: The acute phase protein LBP and, recently, septin, a 90 kDa glykoprotein. We have established a simple in vitro, system for measuring LPS binding to CD14 on human monocytes in MNC-suspensions using FITC-labeled LPS (055:B5) and flow cytometry. Binding of LPS-FITC to monocytes was serum dependent and could be blocked by unlabeled endotoxins or anti-CD14-antibodies, and is not detectable on CD14-negative monocytes. The relation between the concentrations of LBP, septin, soluble CD14 or other interfering LPS-binding serum factors, like HDL, are unknown. Acute phase sera mediate saturating LPS-FITC binding in higher dilutions in comparison to sera of healthy persons. For studying the possible role of soluble CD14, which is able to block LPS-FITC binding to monocytes, as an inhibitor of endotoxic shock it is necessary to quantitate the relation between the effective serum proteins. Serum preparations isolated by ammonium sulphate precipitation, preparative IEF, batch IEC containing LBP or septin, are able to mediate LPS binding to CD14. These results were in agreement with experiments, showing that the opsonizing capacity of whole serum for mediation of LPS-induced oxidative burst response is also mediated by the LBP prepartion alone.

The experiments demonstrate the usefulness of flow cytometry analyzing interactions between supporting and inhibiting factors for endotoxin induced monocyte activation and their consequences.

COMPARATIVE INTERACTION OF GLYCATED AND OXIDIZED LOW DENSITY LIPOPROTEINS WITH HUMAN MONOCYTE-DERIVED MACROPHAGES.

A. GUGLIUCCI CRERICHE, J-C.SIFFERT, S.DUMONT AND A.J.C. STAHL. Département d'Immunopharmacologie, Laboratoire de Biochimie, Faculté de Pharmacie, Université Louis Pasteur. BP 24, F- 67401, Illkirch Cedex, France.

Macrophages play a key role in atherogenesis, being capable of transformation into foam cells, through the uptake of modified LDL. LDL metabolism by human monocyte-derived macrophages (Mϕ) is altered by glycation or oxidation, modifications which could favour atherogenesis in diabetic patients. As glycated LDL (glc-LDL) and oxidized LDL (oxi-LDL) are the only naturally occurring forms of modified LDL, we explored their interaction with Mϕ and compared their stimulation of protease secretion by these cells.

LDL was isolated from healthy human subjects by sequential ultracentrifugation (c-LDL). Glycation was performed by incubation with 50 mmol/l glucose at 37°C during 5 days. Oxidation was carried out by incubation in the presence of 5 μmol/l $CuSO_4$ at 37°C for 20 h. Glycation was measured by a modified fructosamine assay. Thiobarbituric acid reactive substances and lipid hydroperoxides were measured as markers of oxidation. C-LDL, glc-LDL and oxi-LDL were labeled with $Na^{125}I$ according to the Iodogen® procedure. Uptake of ^{125}I-glc-LDL and ^{125}I-c-LDL was studied in cell culture experiments using Mϕ obtained by countercurrent centrifugal elutriation and used after 8 days of primary culture. Competition experiments showed that glc-LDL was able to displace up to 35% of ^{125}I-oxi-LDL at a ten-fold concentration. Conversely, oxi-LDL displaced 45% of ^{125}I-glc-LDL, in the same conditions. Glc-LDL was not significantly oxidized before cell culture experiments. These data show that both oxi-LDL and glc-LDL share a common pathway responsible for the uptake of a fraction of the bulk of added lipoprotein.

Protease secretion by Mϕ was measured using the dye-linked collagen Azocoll®, after stimulation with either c-, glc-, or oxi-LDL. Macrophages were either not treated or previously treated with 10 μg/ml lipopolysacharide (LPS) for 24 h. C-LDL showed a 27% stimulation over basal protease secretion; increment was 80% for glc-LDL and 137% for oxi-LDL. These responses were not significantly different in not treated or LPS-treated Mϕ.

Macrophages have been shown to oxidize LDL, and glc-LDL is reported to be more susceptible to oxidation. In accordance to these facts, one possible explanation to our LDL-uptake results would be that glc-LDL is oxidized during the 5 h-incubation at 37°C and thus it is increasingly recognized by the scavenger receptors. Alternatively, glc-LDL contains a subpopulation of particles sufficiently modified as to become ligands of the scavenger receptors. The differential increment in protease secretion through glc-LDL and oxi-LDL stimulation also support these views. Uptake of a fraction of glc-LDL by Mϕ via this pathway, may contribute to foam cell generation in diabetic patients.

Monocyte Activation and Acute Phase Response in Preoperative Patients

W.Haupt*, C.Pohle*, H.F. Möhring*, N.V. Christou**, W.Hohenberger*

Dpt. of Surgery, University of Regensburg, Germany*
Dpt. of Surgery, McGill University, Montreal, Canada**

Background: Low preoperative serum albumin levels were reported to be associated with postoperative complications. However, sensitivity and specificity of prediction models were low and and additional variables are necessary to improve the model. Furthermore, the reason for a low preoperative serum albumin level is not yet clearly understood. Therefore, we put up the hypothesis, that preoperative serum albumin may be caused by monocyte activation and an subsequent acute phase response.

Study: 164 patients waiting for major abdominal surgery were entered into a prospective study collecting data on preoperative monocyte activation state and acute phase response. Serum neopterin,IL-6, CRP, a-1-antitrypsin, prealbumin and albumin were measured. Malnutrition was ruled out by body composition analysis. Patients with renal insufficiency were excluded (n = 4).

Results: Serum neopterin levels exceeding 10 pg/ml were found in 42.1%. Il-6 could be detected in 15.1 % . Crp levels were raised above 5 mg/dl in 12,0 %, a-1-antitrypsin levels above 350 mg/dl in 18.7 %, prealbumin levels below 10 mg/dl in 7.8 % of all pt´s. Albumin levels below 34 g/l were found in 13.3 % .
66.5% did not have any abnormal values in terms of an acute phase response. However, even in this group of patients raised neopterin levels were found in 33.0%. On the other hand, 40.0% of all pt´s with abnormal acute phase variables had serum neopterin levels below 10 nmol/ml.
Decreased serum albumin levels were associated with other acute phase parameters in 68.2 %. and with raised neopterin levels in 81.8 %.
Presence or absence of an acute phase response was the strongest predictive variable in a logistic regression modell , postoperative septic complication being the variable to predict.

Conclusion: Monocyte activation and an acute phase response were present in a high proportion of preoperative pt´s. However, the data do not suggest a clear cause and effect relationship of monocyte activation and acute phase response. The preoperative regulation of albumin metabolism and mechanisms of preoperative acute phase response need further investigation.

NITRIC OXIDE PRODUCTION AND ADP-RIBOSYLATION IN MACROPHAGES

S. Hauschildt*, P. Scheipers, W.G. Bessler*, P. Mordvintcev+, A. Vanin+ and A. Mülsch#.

* Department of Immunobiology and # Department of Applied Physiology, University of Freiburg, Freiburg, F.R.G.

+ Institute of Chemical Physics, Russian Academy of Science, Moscow, Russia

Murine macrophages contain an inducible Ca^{2+}-independent nitric oxide(NO)synthase which upon stimulation converts L-arginine into citrulline and NO (1). By using electron paramagnetic resonance spectroscopy we show that only NO and not other compounds such as nitrite, hydroxylamine or S-nitrosothiols accounts for the immediate oxygenated species derived from the enzymatic oxygenation of L-arginine. Induction of NO synthase is accompanied by a decrease in ADP-ribosyltransferase activity and a change in the pattern of ADP-ribosylated proteins. Induction can be prevented by inhibitors of poly(ADP-ribose)polymerase. Since the inhibitors suppress protein- , DNA- and RNA-synthesis, they are likely to prevent induction of NO synthase by interfering with these biosynthetic processes.

1. Hauschildt, S., Lückhoff, A., Kohler, J., Bessler, W.G. and Busse, R. (1990) Biochem. J., 270, 351-356.

The Differentiation Pattern of Monocyte-derived Macrophages can still be Influenced by Changes in Culture Conditions

Burkhard Hennemann, Marina Kreutz, Annegret Rehm and Reinhard Andreesen
Klinik und Poliklinik für Innere Medizin I, 8400 Regensburg, FRG

Macrophage (MAC) differentiation from peripheral blood monocytes can be achieved in vitro and different types of MAC are induced by different culture conditions(1). MAC cultured for 7 days in the presence of 2% human serum are characterized by a strong expression of CD14 (88 +/-14% positive cells by flow cytometry), CD16 (49 +/-26% positive cells) and MAX.1 (81 +/-15% positive cells) with 52 +/-16% of initially cultured cells surviving. In contrast, MAC cultured in serum-free medium containing rhM-CSF (100 ng/ml) show a lower expression of these antigens (CD14 37 +/-29%, CD16 10 +/-8%, MAX.1 36 +/-30%) and a cell recovery of 24 +/-10%.
Phenotype and cell survival of mature MAC can still be influenced by changing culture conditions after 7 days of incubation. Serum-cultured MAC reduce antigen expression when consequently cultured in serum-free medium containing rhM-CSF (CD14 57%, CD16 5 +/-6%, MAX.1 36 +/- 26 %. On the opposite, the low expression of these antigens upon cultivation in rhM-CSF containing medium increases after adding serum (CD14 59%, CD16 8 +/-5%, MAX.1 47+/-17%). Cell recovery is decreasing upon replacement of serum-containing culture medium to 28 +/-12% and increasing from 24 +/-10% to 59 +/- 12% upon transferring cells from rhM-CSF to serum.
Similarily a decrease of TNF-secretion of about 30% is seen in serum-cultured MAC upon changing to rhM-CSF medium. Accordingly, TNF-secretion of rhM-CSF-cultured MAC (which is comparable with TNF-secretion of freshly isolated monocytes(1)) is increasing about 70% when culture is continued in the presence of serum.
Therefore, we conclude that differentiation patterns of monocyte-derived mature MAC can still be influenced by the microenvironment of the cells.

1 Kreutz et al, Res Immunol 1992, 143, 107-115

ENHANCED METASTATIC GROWTH IN THE RAT LIVER AFTER SELECTIVE ELIMINATION OF KUPFFER CELLS BY LIPOSOME-ENCAPSULATED DICHLOROMETHYLENE DIPHOSPHONATE.

G. Heuff[1], N. Van Rooijen[2], C.D. Dijkstra[2], S. Meyer[1], R.H.J. Beelen[2].
1 Department of Surgery, Free University Hospital, Amsterdam, The Netherlands
2 Department of Cell Biology, Medical Faculty, Free University, Amsterdam, The Netherlands

Whether Kupffer cells (KC) in vivo are capable in controlling metastatic tumour growth in the liver, is largely circumstantial. In the present study, the effects of selective KC elimination on the occurrence and growth of experimental hepatic metastases has been investigated. Till now, it was not possible to eliminate selectively the KC without affecting other macrophage populations and other cell types, such as lymphocytes. Recently a method has been developed for selective elimination of macrophages to study functional aspects of these cells, using liposome-encapsulated dichloromethylene diphosphonate (Cl_2MDP-liposomes). Intravenous injection of Cl_2MDP-liposomes leads to effective elimination of all KC, without affecting non-phagocytic cells, within 24 hours.
Groups of 8 rats were injected with Cl_2MDP-liposomes, PBS-liposomes (as a control) or a saline solution. Fourty-eight hours later, all rats were inoculated with 10^6 CC531 tumour cells by injection in a mesenteric vein. Two weeks after tumour cell inoculation the rats were sacrificed.
Results show an enhanced metastatic growth in the Cl_2MDP-liposomes-treated group of rats. The livers were almost completely replaced by metastases and increased in weight, whereas in the control groups only a few (4-10) small (1 mm) metastases were found. The tumour load was determined by weighting the livers: Cl_2MDP-liposomes livers weighted 39.4 g (s.d. ± 9.6 g), control livers weighted 10.1 g (s.d. ± 0.9 g; $p < 0.00001$).
In conclusion, these results show clearly that selective elimination of KC with Cl_2MDP-liposomes, results in enhanced metastatic growth in the rat liver. Furthermore these results show that KC play a crucial role in controlling the growth of hepatic metastases. These findings form direct evidence for such a role of KC in vivo.

Cytokine Induced Synthesis from L-Arginine:Implications from Cell-medicated Immunity

John B. Hibbs, Jr., M.D.
Division of Infectious Diseases, Department of Medicine, University of Utah School of Medicine, Salt Lake City, Utah 84132, USA

In 1987, it was reported that expression of inducible activated macrophage cytotoxicity is L-arginine dependent (1). L-arginine is the precursor molecule for an enzyme synthesizing inorganic nitrogen oxides and L-citrulline (2,3). Nitric oxide (NO), a paramagnetic gas with a short half-life, is the inorganic nitrogen oxide that mediates L-arginine dependent cytotoxicity (4,5). The discovery of the L-arginine:NO pathway provided a biochemical explanation for an unusual pattern of metabolic perturbation described previously in tumor target cells of activated macrophages (reviewed in 6) and identified an effector molecule (NO) capable of attacking prokaryotic and eukaryotic intracellular microbes (6). Many intracellular microbes invade and proliferate in cells not specialized for host defense (e.g., endothelial cells, hepatocytes, fibrobalsts, etc.). As a result, the most efficient defense against them is one induced in the cytoplasm of the host cell in which the intracellular pathogen is replicating. The high output NO synthase has been detected in many types of somatic cells (6) and is a soluble cytoplasmic enzyme (5). These are requirements for an efficient defense against intracellular pathogens. Iron nitrosylation is a major biochemical consequence of cytokine induced NO synthesis, suggesting that it may have a role host resistance to intracellular microbes (6).

Interferon- , tumor necrosis factor, and interleukin-1 induce the high output NO synthase in rodent cells (6). High-dose interleukin-2 (IL-2) therapy is known to induce the same cytokines in patients with advanced cancer. Therefore, we examined renal cell carcinoma (RCC; n=5) and malignant melanoma (MM; n=7) patients for evidence of cytokine-inducible NO synthesis. Activity of this pathway was evaluated by measuring serum and urine nitrate (the stable degradation product of NO) during IL-2 therapy. IL-2 administration caused a striking increase in NO generation as reflected by serum nitrate levels (10- and 8-fold increase [P <0.001, P <0.003] for RCC and MM patients, respectively). IL-2 induced renal dysfunction made only a minor contribution to increased serum nitrate levels. Metabolic tracer studies using L-[guanidino-$^{15}N_2$]arginine demonstrated that the increased nitrate production was derived from a terminal guanidino nitrogen atom of L-arginine. These results showing increased endogenous nitrate synthesis in patients receiving IL-2 demonstrate, for the first time, that a cytokine-inducible, high-output L-arginine:NO pathway exists in humans (7).

References:

1. *J Immunol*, 138:550-565, 1987.
2. *Science*,235:473-476, 1987
3. *Proc Natl Acad Sci USA*, 84:6369-6373, 1987.
4. *Biochem Biophys Res Commun*, 157:87-94, 1988.
5. *Biochem*, 27:8706-8711,1988.
6. In Nitric Oxide from L-Arginine: A Bio-regulatory System. S. Moncada&EA Higgs Editors. Elsevier Science Publishers B.V. (Biomedical Division), N.Y. 189-223, 1990.
7. *J Clin Invest*, 89:867-877, 1992.

REGULATION OF TNF-α-mRNA SYNTHESIS IN KUPFFER CELLS IN THE LPS-PERFUSED RAT LIVER: A NON-RADIOACTIVE *IN SITU* HYBRIDIZATION STUDY.

R HOFFMANN, M GREWE, HC ESTLER, A SCHULZE-SPECKING and K DECKER
Biochemisches Institut, Hermann-Herder-Straße 7, D-7800 Freiburg i.Br., Germany

Kupffer cells (KC) in primary culture synthesize TNF-α-mRNA and release mature TNF-α upon stimulation with LPS. Northern blot experiments have shown that transcription is markedly inhibited by PGE_2 and partly by dexamethasone. However, little is known about the ability of individual KC in the intact liver to respond to a LPS challenge and to react *in vivo* in the same way as in primary culture. Although measurements of TNF-α mRNA levels by means of semi-quantitative PCR or Northern blotting allow the assessment of overall TNF-α-mRNA synthesis, they are unsuitable to verify the presence and distribution of specific mRNAs in single cells. We determined, therefore, the presence of TNF-α-mRNA in KC of rat livers that were exposed to LPS, LPS + PGE_2 and LPS + dexamethasone, respectively, applying non-radioactive *in situ* hybridization (ISH) to liver sections.

Rat livers were perfused with RPMI medium containing 100 ng LPS/ml, 100 ng LPS/ml + 1 μM PGE_2, 100 ng LPS/ml + 1 μM dexamethasone and RPMI alone (negative control), respectively, for 90 min. After fixation tissues were routinely processed to paraffin wax. Five μm thick sections were mounted on sterile slides. After proteolysis, *in situ* hybridization of TNF-α-mRNA was carried out overnight at 42°C using digoxigenin-labelled antisense or sense RNA probes generated by *in vitro* transcription. After stringency washes, bound probe was detected by alkaline-phosphatase-conjugated anti-digoxigenin antibody. Size, location and total cell number of detected cells by ISH was compared with KC identified by immunohistochemistry.

With this method we were able to obtain a specific signal in individual cells within the hepatic sinusoids. No signal was detectable in livers perfused with RPMI alone or hybridized with sense RNA. Comparing the location of TNF-α-mRNA-specific signals obtained with the digoxigenin-labelled antisense RNA with that derived from the use of macrophage-specific antibody, a homogenous distribution throughout the liver must be assumed. No indication of a zonal preference was apparent. We conclude, therefore, that all KC, regardless of their anatomical location in the liver, participate in TNF-α-mRNA production after LPS stimulation. Furthermore, it appears that in the perfused liver KC are the only cells in the hepatic sinusoids able to express TNF-α. The number of TNFα-mRNA-positive LPS-triggered KC was reduced in the presence of PGE_2 or dexamethasone. Since the glucocorticoid was found in Northern blot analysis to elicit only incomplete inhibition of TNF-α-mRNA synthesis in KC, an additional regulative process *in vivo* must be considered.

THE ROLE OF INTEGRINS IN MACROPHAGE BIOLOGY

Nancy Hogg, Imperial Cancer Research Fund, Lincoln's Inn Fields, London WC2A 3PX

At present the integrin family consists of 17α subunits and 8β subunits found in 20 heterodimeric combinations (Hynes, 1992). The monocyte/macrophage (Mph) family express a minimum of 10 of these receptors of which only the β2 integrin family (CD11/CD18) of LFA-1, CR3/Mac-1 and p150,95 is restricted to the leukocytes. An inherited lack of expression of CD11/18 causes immune deficiency problems which are particularly the result of impaired myeloid cell function. The integrins participate in Mph functions as diverse as antigen presentation to T cells (Dransfield, et al., 1990), adhesion to endothelium (Hogg, 1992), phagocytosis (Brown, 1991) and recognition of apoptotic neutrophils and T cells (Savill, et al., 1988). The β2 integrins are not constitutively active in terms of ability to bind to ligand and must be stimulated to do so. Integrin-mediated Mph functions, as well as the mechanisms by which integrins are activated will be discussed.

References

Brown, E.J. (1991). Complement receptors and phagocytosis. Current Opinion in Immunology **3**, 76-82.

Dransfield, I., Buckle, A.-M. and Hogg, N. (1990). Early events of the immune response mediated by leukocyte integrins. Immunol. Rev. **114**, 29-44.

Hogg, N. (1992). Roll, roll, roll your leukocyte gently down the vein . . . Immunol. Today **4**, 113-115.

Hynes, R.O. (1992). Integrins: versatility, modulation, and signalling in cell adhesion. Cell **69**, 11-25.

Savill, J., Dransfield, I., Hogg, N. and Haslett, C. (1988). Vitronectin receptor-mediated phagocytosis of cells undergoing apoptosis. Nature **342**, 170-173.

TNF-MODULATION IN CLINICAL STUDIES USING MONOCLONAL ANTI-TNF-ALPHA FOR TREATMENT AND PROPHYLAXIS OF GVHD

E Holler, R Hintermeier-Knabe, B Ertl, E Rustige, M Albiez, M Steimer*, HJ Kolb, W Wilmanns
Med.KlinikIII, Klin.Großhadern, und Inst.f.Klin.Hämatologie, GSF, *Inst.f.Klin.Chemie, Klin.Großhadern, 8000 München 70;

Supported by DFG Grant Ho 1142/1-1

As TNFalpha has been shown to be involved in induction as well as in the effector phase of acute GvHD following allogeneic bone marrow transplantation, phase I/II studies using a monoclonal antibody neutralizing TNFalpha (MAb 195F, provided by KNOLL AG) either for prophylaxis or combined with corticosteroids for treatment of GvHD were started in our unit: In these studies, application of MAb 195F resulted in an unexpected increase of immunological TNFalpha serum levels as determined by different ELISAs: Further analyses revealed that these serum levels are likely to reflect circulation of TNF-anti-TNF-complexes as 1) increase of protein levels was not accompagnied by an increase in TNF bioactivity; 2) immunological TNF-activity could be precipitated by anti-mouse-IgG and 3) TNFalpha release by blood cells seemed to be suppressed during treatment in most patients. These TNF-anti-TNF complexes might visualize tissue production of TNFalpha as indicated by a close negative correlation of absolute levels with dosage of concomitant corticosteroid treatment as well with clinical response of GvHD. In summary, our data suggest that treatment with anti-cytokine antibodies results in changes which are more complex than simple neutralization and elimination of cytokines, and further studies are needed to evaluate the biological significance of cytokine-anti-cytokine complexes.

INTERACTIONS BETWEEN STREPTOCOCCUS MUTANS SEROTYPE POLYSACCHARIDE AND HUMAN MBP.

F. HOLVECK, P. HAAS, L. JUNG, D. WACHSMANN, J. P. KLEIN.
Université Louis Pasteur. Centre de recherches pharmaceutiques.
Département d'Immunologie, Immunopharmacologie et Pathologie. BP 24.
74, route du Rhin. 67401 ILLKIRCH Cedex FRANCE

The human mannose binding protein (MBP), which is synthesized by hepatocytes as a part of the acute response, exists in serum as a multimer of 32 kD subunit and is a member of an ever growing family of animal lectins. Recently it has been established that MBP serves as an opsonin in serum and thereby enhance clearance of mannose rich pathogens by circulating phagocytes. The present work was undertaken to study the interactions between human MBP and a purified serotype polysaccharide prepared from *Streptococcus mutans* OMZ 175 serotype f, a common oral bacterium. The serotype f polysaccharide (poly f) is a rhamnose-glucose polymer having a backbone of rhamnose and side chains composed of terminal alpha linked glucose units.

After purification of the MBP from human sera, by affinity chromatography on a column of Affi-Prep Hydrazide mannan, we demonstrated by Elisa and capillary zone electrophoresis that poly f interacts specifically with MBP. Binding of poly f to the purified lectin is calcium dependent. Upon SDS-polyacrylamide gel electrophoresis, MBP showed, under reducing conditions, two major components having apparent Mr of 70000 and 35000, which interact strongly with biotinylated poly f in Western-blot. We already showed by Elisa, that the specific binding of poly f to human monocytes is significantly enhanced in a dose dependent manner, when poly f is complexed to MBP. These data suggest that MBP could interact with *Streptococcus mutans* via the serotype polysaccharide and experiments are now in progress to assess the relative contribution of human MBP in the physiopathology of some oral streptococci.

DISTINCT IN VIVO FUNCTIONS OF TWO MACROPHAGE SUBPOPULATIONS AS EVIDENCED BY STUDIES USING MACROPHAGE-DEFICIENT op/op MOUSE.

by Wiktor-Jedrzejczak W. Ansari A.A., Szperl M., and Urbanowska E. Dept. Immunology, Central Clin. Hosp., Military School Medicine, Warsaw 00-909, Poland, and Dept. Pathology, Emory Univ. School Medicine, Atlanta, GA 30322, U.S.A.

The op/op mice totally lack macrophage growth factor CSF-1 and thus, by definition are completely depleted of CSF-1 dependent functions of the macrophage cell lineage. Moreover, they possess a severe and generalized macrophage deficiency. However, residual macrophages of these mice should still have normal CSF-1 independent functions. Studies designed to elucidate this issue have revealed that op/op mice are capable of normal in vivo phagocytic function and demonstrate normal humoral and cellular response post immunization with sheep red blood cells. However, release of monokines such as tumor necrosis factor and granulocyte colony stimulating factor following administration of endotoxin is severely impaired in op/op mice as compared with littermate controls. These studies suggest that the CSF-1 dependent macrophage population (absent in the op/op mouse) is primarily responsible for regulatory functions of these cells mediated by monokines, while the CSF-1 independent macrophage population (present in the op/op mouse) is primarily responsible for the classical macrophage functions in immunity such as phagocytosis, antigen processing and presentation.

THE PHAGOCYTIC NADPH-OXIDASE IS EXPRESSED IN THE MONOCYTIC CELL LINE MONO MAC 6

V. Jendrossek, S. Buth, U. Damm, R. Köpp, M. Gahr*
Universitätskinderklinik Göttingen
Robert-Koch-Straße 40, 3400 Göttingen

We analyzed the expression and activity of the superoxide producing NADPH-oxidase normally found in polymorphonuclear leukocytes and monocytes cells in the monocytic cell line Mono Mac 6. This cell line was established from peripheral blood of a patient suffering from monoblastic leukemia with features of mature human phagocytes (H.W.L. Ziegler-Heitbrock et al., 1988).

Mono Mac 6 cells expressed the components of the phagocyte NADPH-oxidase as shown by cytochrome b_{558}-spectrum, FACS-analysis of the cytochrome b_{558} alpha chain and immunoblot analysis of the 47 kDa cytosolic factor. Mono Mac 6 cells reduced nitroblue tetrazolium chloride and produced superoxide after stimulation with different activators of the of the NADPH-oxidase. Preliminary experiments showed that interferon-γ improved superoxide production of Mono Mac 6 cells.

Thus the cell line Mono Mac 6 could serve as model system for the investigation of the inductione of NADPH-oxidase activity in phagocytes by cytokines.

* Supported by DFG-grant Ga 148/7-2

EVIDENCE FOR THE PRESENCE OF RENIN IN MACROPHAGES.

*,+Juillerat-Jeanneret,L.; ;&Corradin-Betz,S.; +Miklossy,J.; +Darekkar,P. *Leuenberger,Ph.; **Division of Pneumology; +Division of Neuropathology; and &Institute of Biochemistry, University of Lausanne, CH 1011 Lausanne, Switzerland*

Angiotensin (Ang) II has been described as a modulator of immune cell functions. Ang II is produced by the sequential action of renin, which is rate limiting and presents 50% homology with cathepsin D, and of angiotensin converting enzyme (ACE). Renin immunoreactivity and ACE activity were examined in human monocytes and bronchoalveolar or brain macrophages, and renin and ACE activities in murine bone marrow-derived macrophages.
Cultured human blood monocytes expressed only cathepsin D and renin expression could not be induced by LPS. Broncho-alveolar macrophages expressed ACE activity and, in distinct cell populations, both renin and cathepsin D. Renin was demonstrated by immunohistochemistry in macrophages accumulating in anterogradely degenerated tracts of human brain. Renin, but not ACE activity, was found in bone marrow-derived macrophages. In these cells, addition of Ang II, but not of LPS, augmented the renin specific activity. These results indicate that products of the renin-angiotensin cascade are specifically expressed in cells of the macrophage lineage and may play a role in their differentiation and activation.

THE ROLE OF MEDIATORS IN THE PATHOGENESIS OF SILICOSIS. II. ISOLATION AND CHARACTERIZATION OF A "FIBROBLAST PROLIFERATION FACTOR" (FPF) FROM QUARTZ DUST-TREATED HUMAN MACROPHAGES

B.Jung, Ursula Thiel, N.H.Seemayer, W. Dehnen, Helga Idel

Medical Institute of Environmental Hygiene at the University of Düsseldorf, Gurlittstr.53, D-4000 Düsseldorf F.R.G.

Quartz dust incubated human macrophages release in vitro a factor, wich stimulates cell proliferation of human lung fibroblasts (Wi-38).

This "fibroblast proliferation factor" (FPF) was classified as a "progression factor". Biological activity of FPF was enhanced in a "complementation test system" with plateled derived growth factor (PDGF) as a "competence factor". In recent studies we could demonstrate, that supernatants of quartz dust treated human macrophages stimulate cell proliferation of human pneumocyte type II cells (line A-549). In our proliferation assay we utilized human pneumocyte type II cells (line A-549). As a proliferation parameter we determined the protein content of cultures after 7 days of incubation. Supernatants of quartz dust exposed macrophages were concentrated by membrane filtration (Amicon centriprep, with nominel molecular weight limit of 10 kDa) and thereafter fractionated by gel-filtration, utilizing Sephadex G 75 and G 150 (Pharmacia). Furthermore, the factor was purified by anion exchange chromatography (Q-Sepharose, Pharmacia). Fractions revealing biological activity in the cell culture test system were further analysed by SDS-gel electrophoresis followed by silver-staining.

By gel-filtration the biological activity of the FPF eluted within a molecular range of 75-102 kD. The active fractions obtained by gel-filtration and anion exchange chromatography showed by SDS-gel electrophoresis two protein bands with apparently molecular masses of 76 and 79 kD, respectively.

A new Hodgkin cell line (HD Zi5) with phenotypic and functional characteristics of mononuclear phagocytes

Ulrich Keilholz, Carmen Scheibenbogen, Thomas Möhler, Kurt Neumann, Ingrun Anton-Lamprecht, Werner Hunstein

Dept. of Medicine (Hematology/Oncology) and Dept. of Dermatology, University of Heidelberg, and Dept. of Pathology, University of Marburg, Germany

Hodgkin and Reed-Sternberg cells have been shown to bear features of both lymphocytes and macrophages, and the origin of this cell type is still a matter of debate. Although phenotypic similarities of Hodgkin cells and macrophages have been demonstrated, functional properties of macrophages have not been examined in great detail in the few Hodgkin cell lines available. We here describe a new Hodgkin cell line resembling macrophages in several phenotypic and functional characteristics. The cell line HD Zi5 has been established in our laboratory from a pleural effusion of a patient with nodular sclerosing Hodgkins` lymphoma. The line continuously grows in RPMI1640, supplemented with 10% fetal calf serum, the doubling time is 2.8 days. The line also continuously grows with 2% human serum instead of fetal calf serum, the doubling time decreases to 4.2 days. Without serum supplement, the cells can only be maintained for several weeks, and the initial doubling time is 10 days. On light and electron microscopy, 80 percent of the cells resemble Hodgkin cells, 20% show the typical features of Reed-Sternberg cells. Pseudopodia, a feature of macrophages not seen in lymphocytes are demonstrated. Cytochemical examination reveals strong reactivity with PAS, a lymphocytic marker, and nonspecific esterase, a monocyte marker. Sudan black, a marker for myeloid cells, is negative. Surface marker analysis with flow cytometry shows high expression of CD71 (transferrin receptor), HLA-DR, and the β-chain of the IL-2 receptor (p75). Expression of CD14 as well as CD13, CD33, and CD10 (CALLA) is also consistently found, and low density CD16 (Fc-Receptor), HLA-I, and CD54. CD71 can be upregulated by IL-1, GM-CSF, and G-CSF, p75 by M-CSF, and HLA-DR by IFN-γ. Constitutive secretion of IL-6, and IL-8 is present, and regulated by many cytokines and lectins. There is no constitutive secretion of Neopterin, but it can be induced by IL-1, IL-6, LPS, and IFN-γ. Release of TNF-α is induced by IL-1, IL-6, and IFN-γ, not by LPS. Another striking feature of this new cell line is the ability for phagocytosis. Latex beads are incorporated, and numerous phagolysosomes can be demonstrated by electron microscopy. In summary, the new Hodgkin cell line shows many characteristics resembling macrophages. These findings contribute to the discussion of the origin of Hodgkin and Reed-Sternberg cells, suggesting close relationship to the lineage of mononuclear phagocytes.

The macrophage response to bacteria and bacterial products.

R. Keller, Immunobiology Research Group, Institute of Immunology and Virology, University of Zurich, Zurich, Switzerland

In a series of studies, the ability of a pure, lymphocyte-free population of bone marrow-derived rat mononuclear phagocytes (BMMø) to respond to heat-killed bacteria and bacterial products was examined. These BMMø were able to respond to these agents with an often marked enhancement of their functional activities, indicating that macrophages do recognize these agents in the absence of components of the specific immune system. Utilizing reduction of MTT, secretion of TNFα and NO/NO_2^-, and expression of TNFα-independent tumoricidal activity as parameters of the macrophage secretory and cellular capacities, the macrophage response to grampositive and gramnegative organisms, to LPS, lipid A, muramyl dipeptide, bacterial oligo- and polysaccharides, peptidoglycans and lipoteichoic acids was comparatively assessed. The findings indicate that the pattern of the macrophage response to a defined bacterial sample is qualitatively similar and readily reproducible; different bacterial agents usually trigger a different macrophage response. Induction of secretory activities and expression of tumoricidal activity were not necessarily associated and were not affected by anti-TNFα, indicating that TNFα is not critically involved in these processes. On the other hand, generation of NO/NO_2^- and expression of tumoricidal activity were suppressed by the flavoprotein inhibitor, diphenyleneiodonium and the L-arginine analogue, NMMA, indicating that induction of the NO synthase pathway is central for the generation of tumor necrosis factor-independent tumoricidal activity by activated macrophages.

Present address: Department of Pathology, Institute of Experimental Immunology, University of Zurich, Sternwartstr. 2, CH-8091 Zurich, Switzerland.

BIOCHEMICAL MECHANISM(S) OF THE MACROPHAGE RESPONSE TO BACTERIAL LIPOPOLYSACCHARIDE (LPS),

T. Kirikae, X. Zhang, F. Kirikae, M-G. Lei and D.C. Morrison. The Cancer Center, Univ. of Kansas Medical Center, Kansas City, KS 66160 USA.

LPS-activated macrophages are capable of killing tumor cells, in large part due to the production of TNF-α and nitroxides (NO). Our efforts to dissect the biochemical pathway(s) for LPS activation of macrophages for tumor cell killing have focused upon identification and characterization of candidate membrane-localized receptors for LPS and mechanism(s) of signal transduction. Using photoactivatable-radioiodinated cross-linking derivatives of LPS, proteins of approximately 80 kDa and 40 kDa have been identified on mouse macrophages and macrophage cell lines. These results have been confirmed using an LPS ligand blotting assay of solubilized and fractionated cell extracts immobilized on nitrocellulose. The available evidence using MAb to the 80 kDa protein suggests that this LPS binding protein can function as a specific LPS receptor for macrophage activation. A mutant cell line (J7.DEF3) reduced in LPS binding, has been isolated from the macrophage cell line J774 which, as assessed by both TNF-α and NO production, manifests altered LPS responsiveness in the presence, but not absence, of serum. The serum-dependent differential responsiveness of parent and mutant has been shown to be critically dependent upon LPS chemotype. Characterization of the mutational defect in the J7.DEF3 cells by photocrosslinking techniques and ligand blotting has suggested that these cells manifest normal levels of 80 kDa and 40 kDa proteins; however, using the ligand blotting assay, a serum-dependent binding of LPS to a protein of 55 kDa is selectively labelled in parental but not mutant cells. Analysis of LPS-dependent signal transduction pathways has implicated a pertussis-toxin (PT) sensitive factor in regulation of LPS-induced TNF-α and NO production. Pretreatment of macrophages with PT, but not PT-B, significantly enhances LPS-dependent TNF-α production but suppresses NO production, suggesting that the production of these mediators is differentially regulated. Further, experiments designed to desensitize macrophages to LPS by pretreatment with subthreshold concentrations of LPS have provided additional support for differential regulation. Thus, LPS pretreated macrophages made refractory to subsequent LPS challenge for NO production are markedly enhanced in TNF-α production and vice versa. Thus, desensitization of macrophages by LPS may actually reflect an LPS-directed selection of a particular biochemical pathway leading to differential macrophage responses. Supported by PO1 CA54474 and R37 AI23447.

LIPOPOLYSACCARIDE (LPS) ACTIVATION OF CD14 ON HUMAN MONOCYTES (Mo) GENERATES PROCOAGULANT ACTIVITY AND INDUCES IL-6 RELEASE.

L.Osnes [1], P.Kierulf [1]., P.Lund [2], Å-B. Westvik[1]
[1]Dept.Clin.Chem.,Ullevaal Univ. Hosp. [2] Fürst Med. Lab.0407-Oslo,Norway

Human cryopreserved Mo may be LPS-instructed to synthezise and express Tissue Factor (TF) resulting in prothrombinase activity, leading to thrombin- and fibrin formation, when exposed to plasma. However, the mechanisms responsible for LPS-activation leading to TF-synthesis is not known. CD14, expressed on the surface of Mo as a glycophosphatidyl-inositol (GPI) -linked protein, is known to be a receptor for complexes of LPS-binding-protein (LBP) and LPS.
AIM: To investigate if CD14 acts as a receptor for LPS-activation of PBM, resulting in IL-6 release, procoagulant activity (PCA) and when exposed to plasma; fibrin formation, (fibrinopeptide A, FPA).
MATERIAL & METHODS: PBM were incubated with a monoclonal antibody to CD14 (Tük4, DAKO), seeded in 5% AT-FCS-RPMI,and LPS-stimulated, the supernatant harvested, IL-6(EASIA;Medgenix) measured and Mo-PCA assessed (chromogenic substrate assay).Separate anti-CD14 PBM-wells were LPS-stiLmulated, offered heparinized plasma, harvested and FPA-appearance assessed. Phosphatidyl-specific phospholipase C (PI-PLC) treated PBM (CD14 removal) were tested as above.
RESULTS & CONCLUSIONS: There was a significant inhibitory effect of anti-CD14 on PCA(80%), FPA(50%) and IL-6 (40%) compared to control cells. Similar results were obtained by PI-PLC treatment. Thus, LPS-activation of human monocytes, resulting in cellular procoagulant activity and IL-6- synthesis and release, appears to be partly mediated through CD14.

SALMONELLA MONOCYTE INTERACTION IN REACTIVE ARTHRITIS.

Juha Kirveskari, Marko Salmi, Sirpa Jalkanen, Kaisa Granfors

National Public Health Institute, Department in Turku, SF-20520 Turku, Finland

Several lines of evidence support the concept that bacterial antigens, especially lipopolysaccharide (LPS), persist in the patients developing reactive arthritis after Salmonella, Shigella and Yersinia infections for longer time than in the patients with uncomplicated disease. First, strong and long persisting antibody responses against the causative agents in sera and synovial fluids of the patients with reactive arthritis suggested the persistence of corresponding antigens. Then, LPS structures were detected in inflamed joints, within mononuclear and polymorphonuclear phagocytes, in patients with Salmonella-, Shigella- and Yersinia-triggered arthritis. It seems likely that the interaction between host and microbe is abnormal and inefficient in HLA B27 positive subjects in whom reactive arthritis develops. In order to evaluate that further, we have recently fed peripheral blood monocytes of healthy people with live Salmonella typhimurium bacteria, and followed expression of certain cell surface antigens during 6-7 days of intracellular life of Salmonella. Despite Salmonella bacteria were living intracellularly, obvious procession of bacteria started in few hours leading to expression of Salmonella antigens on the cell surface. Expression of HLA B27 antigen decreased, and so did other MHC class I antigens in HLA B27 positive cells. Expression of MHC class II antigens DR, DP, DQ seemed to be regulated independently. Expression of CR1 and β_1 -integrins were usually upregulated in HLA B27 negative cells, but downregulated in HLA B27 positive cells. Salmonella bacteria inside the monocytes enhanced the adhesion of these cells on endothelial cell monolayers in vitro. By modulating the surface expression of integrins bacteria inside the monocytes may enhance their binding to synovial endothelium.

BIPHASIC PRIMING OF ALVEOLAR MACROPHAGES FOR ENHANCED RESPIRATORY BURST BY PLATELET-ACTIVATING FACTOR

B.Kleuser, T. Schlüter and G. Gercken

Universität Hamburg, Institut für Biochemie und Lebensmittelchemie, Abt. für Biochemie und Molekularbiologie, Martin-Luther-King-Pl. 6, D-2000 Hamburg 13

The biologically active ether lipid, platelet-activating factor (PAF), which is involved in many inflammatory processes, induces (e.g.) chemotaxis, degranulation, and the release of interleukines and reactive oxygen intermediates (ROI). Furthermore, PAF exerts a priming effect on some cell types. Incubation of polymorphonuclear neutrophils (PMN) with 0.01 to 1000 nM PAF increases the respiratory burst when the cells are challenged by a second stimulus. The activated state occurs immediately after the addition of PAF and disappears after approximately 60 min. In our experiments we studied the priming effect of PAF on cultured bovine alveolar macrophages (BAM). After incubation with PAF over a period from 0 min to 10 h the cells were stimulated by a second agonist. Respiratory burst activity was evaluated by measuring the release of ROI into the incubation medium. A time-dependent biphasic priming was observed: BAM exhibited an enhanced respiratory burst after a preincubation time of 0 to 60 min. In addition, a second maximum of enhanced ROI release could be seen after a priming time of 3.5 to 6 hours. The enhancement of both maximum peaks varied between 15 and 100%, depending on the type of the second agonists, e.g. PMA, concanavalin A, opsonized zymosan, or quartz dust. The lowest effective concentration for PAF priming was 0.1 nM, and maximum values were reached at 100 nM PAF. The specificity of the effect was proven by incubation with lyso-PAF or with PAF and its antagonist WEB 2086. Lyso-PAF was ineffective, and WEB 2086 abolished the PAF priming effect. Thus, the biphasic priming of BAM by PAF seems to be a receptor-mediated process.

Birgit Knepper, Thomas F. Meyer and Jos P.M. van Putten
Max-Planck-Institut für Biologie, Abt. Infektionsbiologie, Spemannstr.34, 7400 Tübingen, Fed. Republic of Germany

Human professional phagocytes: preferred targets for *Neisseria gonorrhoeae* ?

Abstract

Neisseria gonorrhoeae, the causative agent of gonorrhoea, is frequently found intracellularly in human leucocytes and it has been suggested that these cells are a niche enabling *N. gonorrhoeae* to survive the inflammatory response during infection.
We were interested whether the interaction between *N. gonorrhoeae* and human leucocytes is modulated by the expression of variable surface exposed opacity associated proteins (Opa). We therefore performed *in vitro* phagocytosis assays with freshly isolated human neutrophils and monocytes in the absence of serum and examined the dependence of the interaction on Opa expression by microscopy. Interestingly, only OpaC, the Opa-protein which gives rise to an invasive phenotype to epithelial cells (1) was unable to mediate interaction with human neutrophils, whereas the other ten Opa-proteins that can be produced by the same strain increased the interaction rate about ten-fold (2). Remarkably, the association of *Neisseria gonorrhoeae* with human monocytes was Opa-independent, pointing to a different type of interaction with these cells than with neutrophils.
The ingestion and survival of the gonococci inside leucocytes was examined with human monocytes. Infected cells were treated with gentamicin to kill extracellular bacteria and the number of viable intracellular organisms was monitored by colony counting of overnight grown bacteria released from the monocytes by saponin lysis. Our results show that approximately 20% of the initially phagocytosed gonococci survive within monocytes for at least 6 hours. The mechanism underlying this apparent resistance against phagocytic killing is currently being investigated.

References:
(1) S.Makino, J.P.M.van Putten and T.F.Meyer (1991) EMBO J. 10, 1307-1315
(2) E.-M.Kupsch, B.Knepper, I.Heuer, T.Kuroki and T.F.Meyer; in preparation

TUMOR CELLS ELICIT THE RESPIRATORY BURST IN CYTOTOXIC, ACTIVATED BONE MARROW - DERIVED MACROPHAGES (BMDM)

Stephan Körner

Jomol Pharma GmbH, Weissenburgstr. 25, D-8400 Regensburg

Activated macrophages exhibit various cytotoxic and cytostatic activities against tumor cells. To show whether reactive oxygen species (ROS) are involved in cytostasis and antibody independent cytotoxicity, tumor cells were cocultivated with BMDM stimulated with MDP, LPS or an enzymatic digest from *Nocardia opaca* cell walls. Production of superoxide (O_2^-) was followed by Lucigenin enhanced chemoluminescence. Results clearly show that tumor cells are able to elicit the respiratory burst in activated BMDM for several hours whereas no production of O_2^- could be detected with saline treated macrophages. N-acetyl-cysteine, a quencher for O_2^- was used in cytotoxic and cytostatic assays to determine the influence of ROI. It could be shown that O_2^- cooperatively acts with TNF or RNI (reactive nitrogen intermediates) liberated from stimulated macrophages. The respirative burst i.e. production of ROI is a very effective defence mechanism against bacteria and tumor cells and can be enhanced by treatment of macrophages with TNF or the potent immunomodulator interferon-gamma. Both cytokines are produced in large amounts by macrophages and spleen cells, respectively, after incubation with an enzymatic digest from *Nocardia opaca* cell walls. The non toxic extracts from this digest could provide a powerful tool in cancer treatment and are currently under investigation (Jomol®).

DEVELOPMENTAL REGULATION OF VITAMIN D_3-METABOLISM AND VITAMIN D_3 RECEPTOR EXPRESSION DURING DIFFERENTIATION OF HUMAN MONOCYTES

Marina Kreutz[1], Helmut Reichel[2], Stefan W. Krause[1] and Reinhard Andreesen[1]
[1]Klinik für Innere Medizin I, Universität Regensburg and [2]Medizinische Klinik, Sektion Nephrologie, Universität Heidelberg, Germany

The in vitro maturation of blood monocytes (MO) can serve as a model for the in vivo transformation of immature blood MO into macrophages (MAC). Here, when cultured in the presence of serum, MO undergo characteristic changes in morphology, antigenic phenotype and functional activity. We serially measured 1,25-dihydroxyvitamin D_3 (1,25$(OH)_2D_3$) and 24,25-dihydroxyvitamin D_3 (24,25$(OH)_2D_3$) synthesis during in vitro maturation of MO and correlated these functions with maturation-associated changes in the phenotype and secretory repertoire of the cells. The conversion of 25-$(OH)D_3$ into 1,25$(OH)_2D_3$ increased gradually during maturation into MAC. Interferon-gamma augmented baseline 1,25$(OH)_2D_3$-synthesis approximately twofold. The time-course of increased 1,25$(OH)_2D_3$-synthesis correlated with enhanced secretion of neopterin and expression of maturation-associated antigens (MAX.1, CD71). Exogenous 1,25$(OH)_2D_3$ stimulated 24,25$(OH)_2D_3$ synthesis in freshly isolated MO, whereas matured MAC showed no 24,25$(OH)_2D_3$-synthesis. Furthermore, we examined the expression of the vitamin D receptor (VDR). MO constitutively showed a strong expression of VDR mRNA. Differentiation into MAC was accompanied by a marked decrease in VDR mRNA levels. Taken together our results show that MO into MAC differentiation in vitro is associated with (i) an enhanced capacity to synthesize 1,25$(OH)_2D_3$, (ii) a loss of 24,25$(OH)_2D_3$-synthesizing activity and (iii) a decrease in the expression of VDR mRNA. Since 1,25$(OH)_2D_3$ was shown to induce differentiation of MO into MAC, our data suggest an autoregulatory mechanism of MO/MAC generation by 1,25$(OH)_2D_3$.

SECRETION OF PERITONEAL MACROPHAGES TNF-LIKE FACTOR FROM HAMSTERS-BEARING TRANSPLANTABLE MELANOMAS IN RELATION TO BIOLOGICAL PROPERTIES OF MELANOMAS.

Krystyna Kozłowska, Mirosława Cichorek
Laboratory for Cytophysiology, Department of Histology, Medical School, 80-211 Gdansk, Poland

The influence of two kinds of hamster's transplantable melanomas differing in biological properties on the secretion of TNF-like factor by peritoneal macrophages (PM) was studied.

The melanotic melanoma line (Ma) derived from a spontaneous melanoma of the skin and the amelanotic line (Ab) originated from the Ma line by a spontaneous alteration in which loss of pigmentation was accompanied by an acceleration of growth, a greater anaplasticity, changes in the antigenicity and immunogenicity, as well as changes in surface glycoproteins.

The cytotoxicity of 24h cultured PM supernatants on TNF-sensitive cells L929 was measured by using the colorimetric MTT assay according to the method of T.Mosmann et al.

The increase of supernatant cytotoxicity with its concentration has been observed.

In comparison with control supernatant (31±12U/ml or 248±96pg/ml) and of PM obtained from hamsters-bearing Ma melanoma (30±14U/ml or 240±112pg/ml) supernatant of PM obtained from Ab melanoma hamsters-bearing showed a statistically corroborated decrease of TNF-like factor content (14±5U/ml or 112±40pg/ml).

It may be pressumed that differences observed in TNF-like factor secretion by PM may be connected with biological properties of the melanoma lines and reflect the influence of tumor growth on macrophages cytotoxicity.

DETECTION OF LIPOPOLYSACCHARIDE-OUTER MEMBRANE PROTEIN COMPLEXES ON THE SURFACE OF MACROPHAGES USING MONOCLONAL ANTIBODIES IN A TIME COURSE STUDY.

A. Korn[1], H.-G. Kreysch[2], G.A. Luckenbach[2], and K. Nixdorff[1]. [1]Department of Microbiology, University of Darmstadt and [2]Department of Immunopharmacology, E. Merck, 6100 Darmstadt, Germany.

We have shown previously that an outer membrane protein from *Proteus mirabilis* (39 kDa protein) is a very differential modulator of the effects of lipopolysaccharide (LPS) on murine macrophages. Interleukin 1 production by macrophages in response to stimulation with LPS was drastically reduced, while cytotoxicity (tumor necrosis factor production) was greatly enhanced, when the 39 kDa protein was complexed with LPS. In the present investigation, monoclonal IgG antibodies to LPS were used to follow the course of interaction of bone marrow-derived, murine macrophages with LPS and with complexes of LPS and the 39 kDa protein. Macrophages were allowed to react with LPS or LPS-protein complexes for 30 min. Thereafter, they were washed thoroughly and the presence of LPS on the macrophage surface was followed in a modified ELISA over a 24 hour period. When LPS alone was administered, it could barely be detected on the macrophage surface during the assay period. However, the same amount of LPS applied in LPS-protein complexes was readily detectable. At 30 min incubation, LPS appeared in relatively high density on the macrophage surface. Detection decreased thereafter for 4 hours, but reached a new maximum at 24 hours. The results of these assays were confirmed using the Adherent Cell Activated Sorter (ACAS). Measurement of the intensity of fluorescence of single cells indicated that LPS, delivered in complex with the 39 kDa protein, was present in greater density on the surface of macrophages after 24 hours of incubation. The number of cells presenting detectable LPS also increased over this time period.

DIFFERENTIAL DIAGNOSIS OF HYPERCHOLESTEROLEMIA AND RISK ASSESSMENT FOR CORONARY HEART DISEASE BY FLOW CYTOMETRIC ANALYSIS OF MONOCYTES

E. Kovacs, G. Rothe, T. Brüning, G. Schmitz

Institute for Clinical Chemistry, University of Regensburg, Regensburg, F.R.G.

Familial hypercholesterolemia is an autosomal dominant inherited disorder, which results from the genetic defect of the cell surface LDL-receptor. We have established a flow cytometric method with the C7A LDL receptor monoclonal antibody to measure the LDL receptor expression of human monocytes and with Dil-labelled LDL to differentiate between LDL-receptor deficiencies and receptor defects. In our study 384 preselected hypercholesterolemic patients were analyzed with serum cholesterol, LDL, HDL, triglyceride, apo B, apo A-I, Lp(a) levels and apo E polymorphism. In 71,8 % of the patients with cholesterol levels > 300 mg/dl an LDL receptor deficiency was observed and 3 % were found to have a ligand binding- or internalization defect. The immunologic status of circulating monocytes was further characterized as a potential indicator for monocyte involvement in atherogenesis in 46 freshly diagnosed non-treated FH patients. No correlation could be detected between the extent of hypercholesterolemia and the expression of differentiation and activation markers (CD14, CD16, HLA-DR), adhesion molecules (CD11a, CD48, CD58) and membrane bound complement regulatory proteins (CD35, CD46, CD55, CD59). However, patients with coronary heart disease independent of their plasma cholesterol level showed a significantly reduced expression of differentiation and activation markers and membrane bound complement proteins. These results suggest that the flow cytometric analysis of monocytes allows the differential diagnosis of hypercholesterolemia and gives potential parameters for the prognostic assessment of the atherogenic risk and for the development and monitoring of new therapeutical approaches.

N-ACETYL-GALACTOSAMINE SPECIFIC LECTINS REGULATE PRODUCTION OF MACROPHAGES IN RAT BONE MARROW CULTURE.

Walter Krugluger, Marcus Köller, Alois Gessl, Georg Boltz-Nitulescu and Othmar Förster. Inst. of Exptl. Pathology, Univ. of Vienna.

Carbohydrates have been identified as recognition structures in the hemopoietic system. Specific lectin-carbohydrate interactions are supposed to mediate cell-cell and cell-matrix interactions and have been used for the identification and separation of various cell types. Previously we have reported that soy bean agglutinin (SBA) binds weakly to the majority of blast cells in freshly isolated rat bone marrow (BM) but strongly to mature macrophages (MΦ) (W.Krugluger et al., J.Leukocyte Biol. **48**: 451, 1990). Further studies indicate that at least two different SBA-binding structures can be identified: a 26 kDa glycoprotein on freshly isolated BM-cells (BMC) and a 160 kDa glycoprotein on BM-derived MΦ (BMDMΦ). To analyze the functional significance of these glycoproteins BMC were cultured with recombinant murine GM-CSF in the presence or absence of SBA. Presence of SBA (specificity: GalNAc > Gal) in BMC cultures greatly enhanced the proliferation inducing effect of CSF. Pea nut agglutinin (specificity Gal >> GalNAc) had no such enhancing effect. SBA alone did not induce proliferation of BMC. Only the proliferation of committed cells seemed to be stimulated since the number of colonies formed in methyl cellulose cultures was not increased by SBA. However, pretreatment of BMC with GalNAc led to an increase of colony number, which may be caused by a blockade of interaction of hemopoietic cells with an endogenous lectin. Possibly, lectin-carbohydrate interactions may play a role in the regulation of myelopoiesis *in vivo*.

Supported by Austrian Science Research Fund and Anton Dreher Gedächtnisschenkung für Medizinische Forschung.

METHODS OF GENE TRANSFER INTO HUMAN BLOOD MONOCYTES

UTE KREUZBURG-DUFFY & CAROLINE MACDONALD
Department of immmunology, University of Strathclyde, The Todd Centre, 31 Taylor Street, GLASGOW G4 ONR, Scotland.

Normal human peripheral blood monocytes have a finite life-span *in vitro*; the cells have a limited, if any, capacity to proliferate in culture. Attempts to culture fresh normal peripheral blood monocytes for prolonged periods, have met with varying results as to length of culture life and properties of the cells involved. Efforts have been made in our laboratory to develop and optimize techniques for the establishment of long-term human monocyte/macrophage cell lines.

The introduction of viral oncogenes into primary cells is a technique which has been successfully used in order to isolate differentiated mammalian cell lines capable of prolonged or indefinite growth in culture. This technique is known as cell immortalization or establishment and can result in the production of cell lines which retain their original specialised functions during *in vitro* growth. A number of different immortalizing oncogenes exist; among of them the simian virus 40 large T antigen (SV40 transformation or tumour antigen) which is used in our laboratory.

There are various strategies of transferring genes into cells. DNA can be introduced into cells by the formation of a calcium-phosphate precipitate which is then taken up by the cells via endocytosis (transfection); encapsulation of the DNA in liposomes; electroporation; direct microinjection; protoplast fusion and retrovirus-mediated transfer. The former three methods are predominantly used in our gene transfer experiments and will be discussed in detail.

The conditions for efficient gene transfer using each of the methods listed above vary considerably with different cell types and therefore, a wide range of experiments have to be carried out to determine the optimum conditions for highest gene transfer. Modifications in the various transfection protocols as well as different approaches to stimulate the recipient mononuclear cells in an attempt to maximize DNA uptake will be reported.

ENCAPSULATION OF TISSUE FOR TRANSPLANTATION DOES NOT PROTECT FROM MACROPHAGE MEDIATED LYSIS VIA NITRIC OXIDE IN *IN VITRO* EXPERIMENTS

K.-D. Kröncke, F. Wiegand and V. Kolb-Bachofen

Div. of Immunobiology, Dept. of Medicine, Univ. of Düsseldorf, Moorenstr. 5, 4000 Düsseldorf 1, FRG

Type 1 (insulin dependent) diabetes is commonly accepted to be an autoimmune disease. In rat and mouse models many attempts have been made to transplant Langerhans islets into diabetic animals to reverse their diabetic state. To separate the transplanted graft from the host's defence system, the islets are encapsulated in alginate, a polysaccharide gel matrix. After several weeks, the alginate encapsulated transplanted islets are often surrounded by pericapsular infiltrates, the majority of these cells being macrophages and fibroblasts. Viability of encapsulated islets *in vivo* at that time is greatly reduced and thought to be due to malnutrition.

We recently showed that the macrophage secretory product IL-1ß *in vitro* induces lysis of alginate encapsulated islets via endocrine nitric oxide production. We now report that activated but not resident macrophages are able to directly lyse alginate encapsulated islets *in vitro* within 24 h as determined by electron microscopy. Lysis of encapsulated islets is dependent on the target:effector ratio and the L-arginine concentration in the medium. Islet cell lysis can be inhibited by the nitric oxide synthase inhibitor N^G-methyl-L-arginine. Furthermore, nitric oxide, chemically generated by nitric oxide-donors like S-nitroso-N-acetylpenicillamine and SIN-1, mimicked macrophage mediated lysis of alginate encapsulated islets.

We conclude that activated macrophages can destroy transplanted tissue via nitric oxide despite separation by encapsulation in alginate, indicating that the NO radical or an active intermediate are stable enough to allow diffusion into the alginate capsule.

EFFECT OF LPS ON MEMBRANE CD14 IN HUMAN MONOCYTES AND MACROPHAGES

R. Landmann, C. Galanos,[+] and W. Zimmerli, Div. Infect. Dis., Depts. Research and Internal Medicine, University Hospital, CH-4031 Basel, [+]Max Planck Inst. Immunbiology, Freiburg, D.

The membrane form of the 53 kD glycoprotein CD14 is a receptor for LPS, when LPS is bound to the serum factor LBP. The regulation of membrane CD14 (mCD14) after binding of its ligand is unknown. In the present study mononuclear leukocytes (PBL), elutriation purified monocytes or blood monocyte derived macrophages were cultured for 15' to 120' or for 15 to 48h with 0.1 to 100ng/ml LPS (S.typhi, E.coli Re, S.abortus.equi sm). mCD14 was measured by immunofluorescence using the Leu-M3 or the My4 antibody which compete weakly and strongly resp. with LPS for monocyte binding. TNFa was measured by ELISA. LPS did not change monocyte mCD14 during the first two hours of incubation. LPS weakly reduced mCD14 after 15h (10 ng/ml, mean FI:-9±7%), in contrast, it strongly enhanced mCD14 after 48h (10ng/ml:+78±2%). In macrophages this increase of mCD14 appeared already after 15h (10ng/ml:+50±2%). Upregulation reached a plateau at 1 to 10 ng/ml, was similar for the different LPS preparations, for adherent and non adherent cells, and did not occur with another bacterial wall constituent (muramylpeptide). It was similar in cultures with heat-inactivated human AB serum or FCS, but weaker in serum-free cultures. The increase was smaller in PBL cultures (10ng/ml:+47±18%), it was not influenced by anti-IFNg antibodies. Upregulated mCD14 following LPS stimulation coincided with a reduction of the LPS induced TNF response. Potential mediators involved in the LPS effect on mCD14 are being investigated. In conclusion, late mCD14 upregulation may serve to counteract LPS induced adaptation.

PHASE IIa STUDY OF A LIPOSOMAL MURAMYL TRIPEPTIDE IN CANCER PATIENTS: INITIAL PRONOUNCED IMMUNOMODULATORY EFFECTS IN MONOCYTES DECREASE DURING PROLONGED THERAPY

R. Landmann, R. Obrist, H. Denz, C. Ludwig, H. Frost*, M. Wesp*, C. Rordorf*, D. Gygax*, L. Tarcsay*,and J. P. Obrecht, Departments of Research and Internal Medicine, Division of Oncology, University Hospital and *Pharma Division, Ciba- Geigy Ltd.,Basle, Switzerland

Liposomal muramyl tripeptide-phosphatidyl ethanolamine (MTP-PE) was infused in 14 metastatic cancer patients (4mg i.v. during 30 min twice weekly for 12 weeks). Clinical, pharmacokinetic and immunological parameters were studied before and 0.5, 2, 4, 24 and 72h after start of drug infusion in week 1, 4, 8 and 12. No tumor regressions were seen. Tumors progressed in 11 patients, in 4 of them within 2 months; 3 patients had stable disease. The intensity and frequency of side effects (fever and nausea) diminished from week 1 to 12, while the rate of disappearance (24h) of total and free MTP-PE from blood remained unchanged. MTP-PE caused a marked increase of serum TNFa and IL-6 (27-fold and more than 100-fold resp.)in week 1, but not thereafter. It enhanced monocyte HLA-DR and CD14 expression in week 1 and 4, but not at the later time points. In contrast, it caused a persistent,2-fold increase in serum neopterin and young granulocytes (bands) during week 1 to 12. Before therapy, monocyte tumor cytotoxicity and in-vitro monocyte derived TNFa, IL-1ß and IL-6 production were high in 5 patients (group H) and low in 9 patients (group L). Monocyte cytotoxicity and in-vitro cytokine production declined under therapy in group H, Three of the patients in group H had early progression. It was transiently enhanced in week 1 in group L.In conclusion, MTP-PE induced marked immunomodulation; most effects were transient. The reduced incidence of side effects was paralleled by downregulation of monocyte responses, the extent of which was dependent on pretherapy cell activity. An adaptation phenomenon, related to the twice weekly schedule used, may explain the absence of clinical efficacy.

REGULATION OF THE EXPRESSION OF THE LPS-RECEPTOR CD14 BY IL-4 AND IL-6

Roger. P. Lauener, Silke Hüttner, Hans-Peter Hossle and Reinhard Seger
Kinderspital, Steinwiesstrasse 75, 8032 Zürich, Switzerland

CD14 is a monocytic 52 kD glycosylphosphatidylinositol-anchored protein. It has recently been proposed that it serves as a receptor for the bacterial cell membrane component lipopolysaccharid (LPS). Monoclonal antibodies directed against CD14 have been shown to inhibit LPS-induced TNFα-release. LPS is at least partially responsible for the clincal syndrome of gram-negative sepsis, a still often fatal condition. Thus, a better comprehension of mechanisms regulating the expression of CD14 is of great interest in understanding the pathogenesis of LPS-mediated septic shock and a prerequisite for designing rational therapeutic approaches.

We have previously shown that recombinant human IL-4 downregulates CD14. We now have reexamined the role of other cytokines on CD14 expression.

Normal human monocytes purified by adhesion were assessed by flow cytometry for the expression of CD14, CD23 and HLA-DR antigens after stimulation with rIL-6 (100 U/ml) for 48 h. Under baseline conditions, monocytes were 75% $CD14^+$, <5% $CD23^+$, >90% $HLA\text{-}DR^+$. Incubation with rIL-6 did not affect the percentage of CD14 positive cells, but strongly (≥100%) increased the number of CD14 molecules per cell, as indicated by the mean fluorescence intensity (MFI). No change was observed on the expression of CD23 and HLA-DR.

In view of the fact that LPS binds to CD14, our observation that IL-4 downregulates CD14 is consistent with the proposed antiinflammatory effect of this cytokine. The upregulation of CD14 by IL-6 on the other hand is consistent with observations of elevated CD14 levels during acute phase responses in polytraumatized patients. The regulation of CD14 expression by cytokines thus plays a major role in the modulation of the inflammatory response to gram-negative bacteria.

MONOKINE RELEASE BY THP1 CELLS UNDER LPS STIMULATION AS A ROUTINE MODEL FOR HUMAN MACROPHAGE ACTIVATION.

A. Laulan, B. Basuyaux, N. Lepine, J.C.Siffert and J.Bartholeyns
CNTS, 3 Av. des Tropiques, BP 100, 91943 Les Ulis, France.

Human monocytes-macrophages release variable amounts of monokines after LPS stimulation, depending on the blood donor status. We have developped an assay with a human cell line to monitor quantitatively α-TNF release in presence of LPS. THP1 cells activated by γIFN in presence of 10 % FCS in IMDM medium were seeded at 4.10^5 per well in 24 wells plates. LPS was added for 18h in 5% FCS. Supernatants were collected, centrifuged and α TNF level was measured by ELISA. Spontaneous release was between 4 and 6 pg/ml while under LPS stimulation (from 0 to 50 ng/ml), THP1 cells released dose dependently α-TNF in the culture medium (up to 500 pg/ml). This release could be inhibited by anti-LPS antibodies.

This model of α-TNF release by THP1 cells permits reproducible quantification of human monocyte cell activation by endotoxin and can easily be used to evaluate the potency of drugs affecting this process.

TRANSCRIPTIONAL REGULATION INVOLVED IN THE DIFFERENTIATION OF THE HUMAN LEUKEMIA MONOCYTIC CELL LINE, THP-1

LEROY Pascale and AUWERX Johan.
CNRS UMR 134
Centre de Biochimie
UFR Sciences
Parc Valrose
06108 Nice Cedex 2

Our goal is to describe the main regulation processes involved in the differentiation of monocytes to macrophages, mostly at the level of transcription. THP-1, a human monocytic leukemia cell line, differentiates to macrophages when treated with phorbol esters. Differentiated THP-1 cells have many of the characteristics of fully differentiated macrophages. The differentiation process of this monocytic cell line is, so far, the closest to the in vivo process. Because of these characteristics, THP-1 has been developed in our laboratory as a model system in which regulation can be studied during macrophage differentiation of human myeloid leukemia cells (Experientiae, 1991). In order to understand the regulation processes involved during this differentiation, we have followed the expression of different marker genes with an emphasis on oncogenes and genes involved in the metabolism of the lipids. Very early (15-60 min) during macrophage differentiation of THP-1 cells, there is a strong transient transcriptionnal activation of the c-fos and c-jun genes(Nuc. Acids Res., 1990). About 1 hour after the start of differentiation of these cells, a 15-fold transient increase in LDL-receptor and HMG-CoA reductase trancripts is found. The increase in LDL-receptor mRNA is caused by enhanced transcription, while for HMG-CoA reductase, there is both enhanced transcription rate and increased stability of the mRNA. Furthermore, a new mechanism for regulation of the LDL-receptor gene transcription, on the top of the feedback regulation by cholesterol (described previously by Brown and Goldstein), was delineated. With the use of cycloheximide, it was demonstrated that the LDL-R gene is under the influence of a labile negative trans-acting factor (Proc. Natl. Acad. Sci. USA, 1989). Later during differentiation of THP-1 cells, transcription of the LPL, ApoE and Scavenger receptor was increased. This feature of THP-1 cells is remarkable, since in several of the other studied cell lines (HEL, HL60, U-937) none of these genes are detectable after differentiation to macrophages (Biochemistry, 1988,1989) At present we are analysing the regulartory sequences of several of these genes. Special attention will be paid to the labile negative trans-acting protein involved in repression of the LDL-R gene.We are currently studying LDL receptor and Scavenger receptor promoters as, respectively, an early and a late marker gene in order to isolate transcription factors important for the differentiation process.

Auwerx J.H. (1991) Experientiae 47, 22-31.
Auwerx J.H., Chait A., Deeb S.S. (1988) Proc. Natl. Acad. sci. USA 86, 1133-1137.
Auwerx J.H., Deeb S., Brunzell J.D., Peng R., Chait A. (1988) Biochemistry 27, 2651-2655.
Auwerx J.H., Deeb S., Brunzel J.D., Wolfbauer G. and Chait A. (1989) Biochemistry 28, 4563-4567.
Auwerx J.H., Staels B., Sassone-Corsi (1990) Nucl. Acid Res. 18, 221-228.

EFFECT OF ADENOSINE ON TNF PRODUCTION

V. Le Vraux, Y.L. Chen, I. Masson, M. De Sousa, I. Florentin, J.P. Giroud and L. Chauvelot-Moachon.
Department of Pharmacology. CNRS URA 595. Bat. Roussy, Hôpital Cochin, 27 rue du Faubourg Saint Jacques. 75674 Paris - France.

Adenosine is a ubiquitous modulator of cellular functions which regulates energy/supply demand balance. It acts on membrane-bound receptors (mainly subtypes A_1 and A_2). Its properties are characterized by a decreased release of neurotransmitters, antiarrythmic effect and relaxation of smooth muscle. It also presents antiinflammatory and immunoregulatory activities. In particular, adenosine and its more stable analogs can inhibit adjuvant-induced arthritis, reduce the severity of carrageenan-induced pleurisy in rats and inhibit superoxide anion generation by neutrophils. We tested the hypothesis that adenosine may act, at least in part, via a down-regulation of tumor necrosis factor (TNF) using endotoxin-stimulated human monocytes in vitro and rats receiving a sub-letal dose of endotoxin.

Adenosine and five other receptor agonists were tested. They inhibit TNF production by endotoxin-stimulated monocytes in a concentration-dependent manner. The rank order of agonist potency suggested the involvement of the A3 receptor subtype described by Ribeiro and Sebastio. The active concentrations of adenosine (IC50 value = $0.82 \pm 0.11 \times 10^{-6}$ M; mean ± SEM; n = 3 different cell donors) are physiologically relevant. Phenylisopropyladenosine (R-PIA) was found to be the most potent with an IC 50 value of $0.35 \pm 0.09 \times 10^{-6}$ M (n = 4). Similar TNF inhibition was obtained by immuno- and bioassays. The effect of R-PIA was predominant on TNF with a slight reduction of IL1β concentrations and no modification of IL6 (tested on B9 cells). TNF inhibition by R-PIA was in part abolished by an antagonist of adenosine receptor. Dipyridamole which inhibits cellular uptake of adenosine and, thus, increases pericellular concentrations of the mediator, had the same effect on cytokine production by monocytes. Finally, pretreatment of rats by R-PIA before endotoxin injection reduced serum TNF levels from 47,500 ± 6,812 U/ml (endotoxin group) to 1000 ± 124 U/ml (R-PIA + endotoxin group) with no modification of IL6 concentrations.

We conclude that TNF inhibition could be an important mechanism by which adenosine analogs exert their antiinflammatory effects.

CLONING AND EXPRESSION OF A HUMAN MONOCYTE/MACROPHAGE ANTIGEN DETECTED BY THE MONOCLONAL ANTIBODY Ki-M1P

R. Lilischkis, A. Salmassi, F. Zschunke*, K. Heidorn, K.Jaquet, H. Heidebrecht, H. Kreipe, M.R. Parwaresch and H.-J. Radzun*
Institute of Pathology, University of Kiel, Michaelisstraße 9, 2300 Kiel, *Institute of Pathology, University of Göttingen, Robert Koch Straße 40, 3400 Göttingen

The cloning of the antigen recognized by a new monoclonal antibody, designated Ki-M1P, is described. Ki-M1P recognizes, in particular, monocytes and different macrophage subsets. The recognized antigen is localized mainly in vesicular structures of the cytoplasm. Since the Ki-M1P antigen is preserved during routine formalin fixation followed by paraffin embedding of tissues, it represents a useful diagnostic tool for the identification of monocytes and macrophages even in archival material.

Using a cDNA library of the monocytic cell lineage THP-1, a 1767 base pairs DNA fragment was isolated by antibody screening. Subcloning in E.coli expression systems resulted in expression of a single 40 kDa protein displaying the Ki-M1P epitope. The cDNA contains polyadenylation signals, as well as a poly A tail; however, the 5' end of the coding open reading frame is truncated. Northern blot hybridizations with this cDNA uncovered a 3 kb transcript in human alveolar macrophages.

In comparison to the immunoprecipitation results from macrophages yielding a 60 kDa protein, it is presumed that the isolated cDNA is a 5' truncated version of the native 3 kb transcript. Sequence comparisons did not reveal significant homology to known genes. We conclude that Ki-M1P represents a new monocyte/macrophage specific differentiation antigen.

COLLECTION OF CIRCULATING MONOCYTES MOBILIZED IN VIVO BY GM-CSF IN CANCER PATIENTS AND SUBSEQUENTLY CULTURED IN VITRO WITH GM-CSF ALLOW THE PRODUCTION OF LARGE AMOUNTS OF MACROPHAGES FOR ADOPTIVE IMMUNOTHERAPY TRIALS. M. Lopez , C.Louvet, C. Martinache, F. Scotto, V. Smadja, C. Mathiot, F. Beaujean, A. de Gramont- Inserm U76, CNTS, Paris - Médecine Interne-Oncologie, Hopital Saint-Antoine, Paris - CDTS du Val de Marne, Créteil - Service d'Hématologie , Institut Curie, Paris.

In a previous pilot study of adoptive transfer of activated autologous macrophages performed in 12 cancer patients (1), a mean reinfusion of 0.28×10^9 macrophages per cycle was very well tolerated and no toxic limiting cell dose was attained. Based on the rationale that increased numbers of macrophages would result in increased antitumoral responses, our efforts were focused on obtaining larger amounts of macrophages available for reinfusion into patients. We first improved the culture conditions to increase the macrophage yield, i. e. the number of seeded monocytes which differentiate into macrophages. The best culture conditions were defined as seeding of mononuclear cells (as previously described by Andreesen et al (2)) in Teflon bags with a high air-liquid surface exchange and in presence of GM-CSF. Our goal was then to increase the number of circulating monocytes in patients with injection of GM-CSF, and to collect higher numbers of monocytes to be seeded. In order to evaluate the faisability of such a procedure, we performed a pilot study in 2 patients. Both presented a metastatic colorectal cancer refractory to 5 FU- folinic acid treatment. Seven leucapheresis were performed to collect leucocytes. The first one (day 1) was performed before in vivo GM-CSF administration and resulted in collection of 11.8 and 5.9×10^9 leucocytes for pts 1 and 2 respectively. Pts then received GM-CSF (Schering-Plough) subcutaneously (5mg/kg/day) from day 1 to day 14 and from day 24 to day 37. Leucocyte counts increased to a mean of $45 \times 10^3/mm^3$. The remaining leucapheresis were performed on days 8, 11, 15, 30, 34 and 38 They resulted in a mean collection of 17.1×10^9 and 12.8×10^9 leucocytes for pts 1 and 2 respectively. MNC were cultured for 7 days in Teflon or Lifecell bags with IMDM supplemented with 2% autologous serum and 500 U/ml GM-CSF.. IFNg (250 U/ml) was added to the culture 18 hours before macrophage harvesting. Activated macrophages were separated from other cells by elutriation. After in vivo GM-CSF treatment, the mean number of macrophages harvested per culture was 2×10^9 (range 1.3 - 2.6) and 2.4×10^9 (range 1.8-3.1) for Pts 1 and 2 respectively as compared to $0{,}6 \times 10^9$ and $0{,}2 \times 10^9$ after culture of MNC collected without GM-CSF mobilization. The activated macrophages were reinfused intravenously to the patients. No chills, no fever and no other side effect were observed upon the 14 reinfusions. In conclusion , this pilot study demonstrated that administration of GM-CSF to cancer patients allows the recovery of large amounts of monocytes which after in vitro culture with GM-CSF generates high numbers of macrophages available for adoptive immunotherapy trials.

(1) Lopez et al, J.Immunotherapy 1992, 11:209
(2) Andreesen et al, Cancer Research 1990, 50:7450

Production of IFN γ activated monocyte-derived macrophages from leucapheresis products of normal donors Analysis of the culture parameters and improvement of macrophage yield with GM-CSF, M-CSF and IL-3.. M. Lopez, C. Martinache, S. Canepa, M. Chokri, J. Bartholeyns, F. Scotto - Inserm U76, Centre National de Transfusion Sanguine, Et Saint-Antoine, Paris - CRTS, 37-Tours - CNTS, Les Ulis.- CDTS du Val de Marne, 94-Créteil.

Blood monocytes collected by apheresis from healthy donors were differentiated in vitro to macrophages which were subsequently activated with rh-gamma interferon. Seven days cultures were performed by seeding Ficoll-separated mononuclear cells or elutriation-purified monocytes under different culture conditions. The best macrophage yields required the seeding of mononuclear cells (instead of purified monocytes) in Teflon bags with a high air-liquid surface interface. The effects of GM-CSF, IL3 and M-CSF on the macrophage yield were then evaluated. GM-CSF increased the average yield by 3.6 and 2.3 fold when purified monocytes or total mononuclear cells were seeded respectively . The corresponding increases with IL-3 were 2.5 and 2.1 fold respectively and with M-CSF 1.2 and 1.4 fold respectively. Macrophages matured under these various conditions displayed similar CD14, CD64, CD71, HLA-DR and Max 1 antigen expression and similar in vitro antitumoral activity against U937 cells. This technique of culture in presence of cytokines allows a large scale production of activated macrophages for adoptive immunotherapy trials.

THIAZOLO-ISO-INDOLINONES, A NEW CLASS OF NON-NUCLEOSIDE HIV-1 REVERSE TRANSCRIPTASE INHIBITORS AND THEIR EFFECTS IN HUMAN PERIPHERAL BLOOD MONONUCLEAR CELLS

Maass G.(1), Koenig B.(2), Leser U.(2), Mertens A.(2) and Pfaff E.(1)

(1) University of Tuebingen, D-7400 Tuebingen, FRG
(2) Boehringer Mannheim GmbH, D-8122 Penzberg, FRG

Selective inhibitors of HIV reverse transcriptase (RT) were identified in a high efficiency screening system, containing purified HIV-1 RT (expressed in E.coli), an in vitro transcript of HIV-LTR including the primer binding site as template and an 18mer oligonucleotide as primer. Inhibition of RT was determined by a non-radioactive RT-assay (ELISA).

Inhibitory compounds were further analysed for their biological activity in HIV infected cell culture. Assays were performed in human peripheral blood lymphocytes and human macrophages. Several HIV-1 isolates (including an AZT-resistant isolate) as well as a HIV-2 isolate were used.

A chiral structure with high specificity towards the RT of HIV-1 was identified with BM 21.1298, a thiazolo-iso-indolinone. The most potent derivatives of BM 21.1298 inhibited HIV-1 RT with IC50-values of 20-100 nM. Results from cell culture assays show similar IC50 values and high specifity for HIV-1. No antiviral effect was noticeable with the HIV-2 isolate. BM 21.1298 was equally effective with an AZT-resistant HIV-1 isolate.

Thiazolo-iso-indolinone resistant isolates of HIV-1 were generated in different cell culture systems. Amino acid changes in the RT-gene of HIV-1 leading to viral resistance were localized.
In another approach, chimeric HIV-1/HIV-2 Reverse Transcriptase mutants were constructed by oligonucleotide-directed mutagenesis. HIV-2 RT substituted with amino acids 179-190 from HIV-1 RT acquires partial sensitivity to BM 21.1298.

ROLE OF 27E10 ANTIGEN IN MACROPHAGE CYTOSKELETON ASSOCIATION AND ADHERENCE

Karsten Mahnke, Ranjit Bhardwaj and Clemens Sorg
Institute of Experimental Dermatology, University of Münster, D-W-4400 Münster, Germany

Appearance of 27E10 epitope-bearing macrophages characterize exclusively acute inflammation. The 27E10 antigen is a non-covalently linked heterodimer of two calcium-binding proteins MRP8 and MRP14, both belonging to the S-100 protein family (1,2). The antigen shows, in a calcium-dependent manner, an increased cell-surface expression.
We further analyzed intracellular distribution and association of this antigen with cellular components.
Confocal laser scan microscopy demonstrated association of the antigen with cytoskeleton. This could be confirmed biochemically. Moreover, we asked whether 27E10 antigen plays a role in mediating adherence mechanisms, which are not well known for macrophages. Adherence of unstimulated macrophages on fibronectin or laminin-coated dishes could be blocked (30%) by 27E10 monoclonal antibody. This inhibition is of the same order of magnitude as compared to that obtained (40%) by antibodies against CD11 and CD18.
We conclude that the 27E10 antigen is involved in regulation of monocyte motility and in mechanisms of macrophage recruitment, particularly those with acute inflammatory phenotype.

1 Bhardwaj, R., C. Zotz, G. Zwadlo-Klarwasser, J. Roth, M. Goebeler, K. Mahnke, M. Falk, G. Meinardus-Hager, C. Sorg: Eur. J. Immunol. 1992, 22, 1891.
2 Zwadlo, G., R. Schlegel, C. Sorg: J. Immunol. (1986) 137, 512.

DO ADENOSINE (ADO) AND CHLOROADENOSINE (CADO) MODULATE LYMPHOPROLIFERATIVE RESPONSES THROUGH AN ACTION ON MACROPHAGES?

I. Masson*, V. Le Vraux*, J. Mathieu**, B. Chanaud*, M. De Sousa*, S. Strzalko*, L. Chauvelot-Moachon*, J.P. Giroud* and I. Florentin*.
* Département de Pharmacologie (URA CNRS 595), Hôpital Cochin, Paris. **Département de Radiobiochimie, Centre de Recherche du Service de Santè des Armées, La Tronche, France.

We have demonstrated that adenosine analogs directly act on monocytes, inhibiting TNF production (Le Vraux et al, abstract in the same issue). In the present work, we investigated whether ADO and CADO could affect proliferative responses of spleen cells from normal and immunodepressed animals (burn-induced immunosuppression).

When acting on normal mouse spleen cells, ADO (in presence of an adenosine deaminase inhibitor) and CADO inhibited proliferative responses to T cell mitogens in a dose-dependent manner with a IC_{50} of 10^{-4} and 10^{-6}M respectively. However, the mechanisms of action of these two drugs seem different. CADO appears to act through a toxic effect on macrophages, already described by Ohtani et al.(1982) and Saito et al (1985), evidenced, in our hands, by a decrease of cell viability and of nitric oxide.production capacity (peritoneal macrophages and J774 cell line). Moreover, CADO immunosuppressive effect was non reversible and was not alleviated by A1 and A2 receptor antagonists.

Thermal injury in rats induced a marked depression of lymphoproliferative responses to T cell mitogens. ADO and CADO fully restored these responses at 1×10^{-5} and 5×10^{-7} M respectively. The question arises whether this immunorestorative effect is related to an action on macrophages. The following observations support this hypothesis : a) the elimination of macrophages from the spleen of burned rats restored the mitogenic responses; b) besides to its own restorative effect, ADO abrogated the one of CADO by protecting macrophages from CADO toxicity ; c) ADO and CADO increased cAMP levels in macrophages (Saito et al). Spleen cell treatment with agents known to elevate cAMP also restored their reactivity to mitogens.

These results strongly suggest that macrophages are the target cells for the immunomodulatory activity of ADO and CADO and are responsible for burn-induced immunodepression.

A L-ARGININE-DEPENDENT METABOLISM IS INVOLVED IN THE CONTROL OF THE TRYPANOSOMA CRUZI INFECTION BY INTERFERON-GAMMA ACTIVATED MACROPHAGES.

METZ G., Y. CARLIER, and B. VRAY. Laboratoire d'immunologie, Université Libre de Bruxelles, 1070 Bruxelles, BELGIUM.

Nitric oxide, derived from the L-arginine catabolism, is thought to be implicated in the control of a variety of infectious microorganisms. By inhibiting the nitric oxide synthesis, we show clearly that the impairement of the Trypanosoma cruzi infection by the gamma interferon-activated murine peritoneal macrophages, is depending on the L-arginine catabolism. The nitrite production by activated macrophages is enhanced when the oxygen-dependent metabolsm in inhibited, indicating an interdependance between these two metabolisms. This nitrite production is also enhanced when activated macrophages are infected with the parasite.

THE ROLE OF MACROPHAGES IN EXPERIMENTAL LYME BORRELIOSIS

M.Modolell, U.Schaible, I.Corraliza[1], M.Rittig[2] and M.M. Simon. Max-Planck-Institut für Immunbiologie, Stübeweg 51, 7800 Freiburg,FRG [1])Depto. de Bioquímica, Facultad de Veterinaria, Universidad de Extremadura, 10071 Cáceres, Spain and [2])Departament of Anatomy University of Erlangen, Erlangen, FRG

Lyme Borreliosis (L.B.) is a tick-transmitted infectious disease caused by the spirochete *Borrelia burgdorferi (B b.)*. In previous studies in a mouse model for L. B. we have found that in contrast to many inbred mouse strains immunodeficient (SCID) mice develop a persistent spirochetemia and chronic arthritis, myositis, carditis and hepatitis. As the majority of the infiltrating cells found in the inflammatory lesions of this mice were identified as Mac-1 positive cells we have studied the role of macrophages in *B.b.* infection. To determine spirochetocidal activity of murine bone-marrow derived macrophages (BMMØ), an *in vitro* system based on the release of radioactivity from prelabeled and killed spirochetes has been established. Furthermore different effector functions of BMMØ were analyzed. The results show that: a) naive BMMØ of all strains tested (BALB/c, C57Bl/6, CBF1, AKR, C.B-17, C.B-17-SCID) are able to kill the spirochetes; b) *B.b.* triggers the induction of O_2^-, NO, TNF and arginase, the expression of class I and class II as well as tumor cytotoxicity; c)IFN-γ further increases the synthesis of O_2^- and NO but not the phagocytosis and kill of *B.b.*; d) opsonisation of the spirochetes with mAbs against the outer surface proteins A and B (OspA, OspB) but not against flagellin increases the induction of O_2^- and NO as well the phagocytosis and kill of the microorganisms; e) inhibition of synthesis of O_2^-, NO or both by superoxide dismutase or N-monomethyl-arginine respectively, leads to reduction but not total abrogation of the killing potential; and f) treatement with chloroquine or cytochalasine B reduces the spirochetocidal activity of BMMØ. These results indicate that MØ use a multiple mechanism to phagocytose and kill. As SCID mice develop spirochetemia and chronic disease in spite of the presence of fully competent MØ, the data indicate that a specific immune response, in particular antibodies against OspA and OspB are necessary for complete eradication of spirochetes from the host. Furthermore, the results suggest that interaction of spirochetes with macrophages is responsible for the induction of the chronic inflamatory disease in these mice.

TROPHIC ACTION OF N-HEXACOSANOL (C26-OH), A LONG-CHAIN SATURATED FATTY ALCOHOL, ON MURINE MACROPHAGES.

I. Moosbrugger (1), P. Bischoff (1), B. Luu (2), J. Waler (3) and J. Borg (4)
(1) Institut d'Hématologie et d'Immunologie, STRASBOURG (FRANCE) ; (2) CNRS URA 31, STRASBOURG (FRANCE) ; (3) Institut de Parasitologie, STRASBOURG (FRANCE) ; (4) MEDAFOR, ILLKIRCH (FRANCE)

N-hexacosanol (ceryl alcohol) is a long-chain saturated alcohol extracted from *Hygrophila erecta*, a plant used in some asian countries for the healing of external wounds. In animal kingdom, C26-OH represents the major component of *spermaceti*, a galenic preparation obtained from the "white horse" found in the whales heads. It is also synthetised by the brain during development. We previously reported that this fatty alcohol, at 500 nM, has a potent differentiating effect on cultured neurons (Borg et al, FEBS Lett., 213, 406-410, 1987) and that it is able to promote, in the rat, the survival of damaged septal cholinergic neurons (Borg et al, Brain Res., 518, 295-298, 1990). In cultured macrophages, C26-OH, at 20 µM, induces several morphological changes and increases their phagocytic capacities. These effects do not reflect an activation process, since neither production of IL-1 or TNF alpha, nor modifications of the MHC class II expression can be observed. (Moosbrugger et al, Int. J. Immunopharmac., 14, 293-302, 1992). C57BL/6 mice were given C26-OH intraperitoneally or per os, (at doses ranging from 10 to 40 mg/kg) and their phagocytic activity was tested *ex vivo* and *in vivo*, using *Saccharomyces cerevisiae*. A 140 % and 50 % increase in the number of yeast/cell was recorded in *ex vivo* and *in vivo* experiences respectively, as compared to controls. These results suggest that this compound may be particularly useful to promote the phagocytic function of macrophages during infection. We are presently investigating the ability of C26-OH-treated mice to resist an infection by *Candida albicans*.

EXPRESSION OF THE FORSSMAN GLYCOSPHINGOLIPID ANTIGEN ON MURINE BONE MARROW-DERIVED MACROPHAGES IS MODULATED SPECIFICALLY BY LYMPHOKINES OF T_H2-CELL ORIGIN

David A. Monner and Peter F. Mühlradt. Gesellschaft für Biotechnologische Forschung, Mascheroder Weg 1, 3300 Braunschweig.

The Forssman (Fo) antigen is expressed on distinct subpopulations of murine macrophages both in vivo and in vitro. In addition, Fo expression on bone marrow-derived macrophages (BMDM) is subject to an age-dependent regulation, increasing from less than 10% Fo+ cells during the first two weeks of culture to a maximum of 50%-60% Fo+ cells during the third week. IL-4 and IL-6 were found to induce an earlier increase in this Fo+ fraction. We now show that the premature induction of the Fo marker on BMDM is specifically regulated by lymphokines derived from the T_H2 cell subclass. BMDM, grown under serum-free conditions, were induced for 48 hr with lymphokines at successive two-day intervals. Antigen expression was assayed using a whole cell ELISA. Premature Fo expression was induced on BMDM by the T_H2-specific lymphokines IL-10, IL-6 and IL-4 in that order of potency, but not by IL-2 or IFN-γ, which are both T_H1-specific. Of the lymphokines produced by both T_H classes, GM-CSF was a potent inducer of Fo whereas TNF and IL-3 were inactive. The modulation was specific for Fo, as expression of the macrophage markers Mac-1 (C3bR), F4/80 and ER-BMDM-1 was not affected by any of the lymphokines. MHC class II expression was induced only by IFN-γ and to a lesser extent by GM-CSF and thus did not appear to be coordinated with expression of Fo. These findings, together with our earlier observation that Fo+ macrophages are localized in the T-cell areas of spleen and lymph nodes, may suggest a discrete role for the Fo+ macrophage in T-cell interactions.

COMBINED INFLUENCE OF OZONE, NO_2 AND PARTICLES ON THE CYTOKINE RELEASE BY MACROPHAGES

M. Mosbach, G. Polzer, A. Seidel

Kernforschungszentrum Karlsruhe, Institut für Genetik und Toxikologie, Postfach 3640, D-7500 Karlsruhe 1, Germany

Ozone and NO_2 are widespread air pollutants. Especially ozone has an influence on lung function in relatively low concentrations. In normal life, man is exposed to a combination of gases and particles, which are primarily deposited in alveolar macrophages after inhalation. The aim of our study was to identify the contribution of the reaction of alveolar macrophages to the general effects of the gases and to look for possible synergistic effects of particles plus gases. For these experiments a special exposure system was chosen, which allowed a direct exposure of the cells in the gas phase. The experiments were performed with human (HAM) or bovine alveolar macrophages (BAM) and calcitriol-differentiated HL-60 cells (HL-60-M), which resemble macrophages in many respects. After LPS stimulation they produce TNFα, IL-6, IL-8 and after Zymosan stimulation superoxide anion.

HAM, BAM and HL-60-M were exposed in vitro to ozone in concentrations from 0.2 to 2.5 ppm for 2 hours. The release of cytokines was analyzed after a 4 h incubation period after the end of ozone exposure. The viability of the HAM and BAM remained normal up to 2.5 ppm whereas the viability of the HL-60-M was reduced to 70% of control by 0.5 ppm ozone. In HAM and BAM ozone induced a concentration-dependent release of TNFα and of a chemotactic factor (ChF) for alveolar macrophages and neutrophils. HL-60-M cells could not be stimulated to a release of TNFα by ozone but they released IL-8, IL-6 and ChF. This ChF is not identical with IL-8, but possibly is C5a. The phagocytosis of quartz (50 µg/ml) induced a release of all of the investigated cytokines whereas latex (250 µg/ml) was biological inert. There were no synergistic effects of a combination of ozone with quartz or latex.

In contrast to ozone, there was no production of IL-6 or IL-8 by HL-60-M after exposure to NO_2 (1 h, 3 ppm), also TNFα was not released. With the exception of IL-6, a preexposure of HL-60-M to NO_2 has a distinct inhibitory effect on the stimulus induced release of the mediators. As with ozone, there was no synergistic effect of latex and NO_2.

The results show that ozone is a potent inducer for the release of proinflammatory mediators whereas NO_2 can inhibit their stimulus induced production. Several clinical findings can be explained by these observations. Possible species differences in the response of TNFα need further evaluation. It can be concluded that macrophages play an important role in the reaction of the lung not only to particles but also to gases and that there is no synergistic effect between both agents.

This work was supported by the project "Environment and Health" (PUG), Kernforschungszentrum Karlsruhe.

Developmental Expression of Leukotriene Metabolizing Enzymes and Leukotriene Binding Proteins on Human Monocytic Leukemia Cell Lines

Thomas Möhler*#, Wolfgang Hagmann*, Michael Müller* and Dietrich Keppler*
*Deutsches Krebsforschungszentrum, Division of Tumor Biochemistry, #Department of Medicine (Hematology/Oncology), University of Heidelberg.

Cysteinyl leukotrienes are biologically potent lipid mediators of inflammatory processes. At the site of inflammation macrophages and monocytes are an important cellular source of leukotriene biosynthesis.

In our study the activity of cysteinyl leukotriene-metabolizing ectoenzymes (γ-glutamyltransferase and LTD_4 dipeptidase) on the human monocytic leukemia cell lines HL60 and U937 were investigated with respect to their state of differentiation.

The conversion of LTC_4 to LTD_4 by γ-glutamyltransferase was readily detectable on both cell lines showing a rate of conversion of 2.5 pmol/10^6 cells within 4h. While U937 cells had an activity to convert LTD_4 to LTE_4 by LTD_4 dipeptidase in the same range as their γ-glutamyltransferase activity, on HL60 cells the rate of conversion of LTD_4 to LTE_4 was detected to be only 0.2 pmol/10^6 cells within 4 h. Differentiation of HL60 cells with 1.25 % DMSO induced a 5-fold increase in their LTD_4 dipeptidase activity and a 1.3-fold increase in their γ-glutamyltransferase activity.

Additional studies using photoaffinity labeling with leukotrienes showed that specific and significant labeling of [^{3}H]LTD_4-binding proteins was only detected in the cellular membrane of DMSO-differentiated, non-proliferating HL60-cells. The apparent relative molecular masses of these LTD_4-binding proteins were 54000, 47000, and 43000.

These studies indicate that malignant, undifferentiated myelo-monocytic cells show only partial expression of cysteinyl leukotriene-metabolizing ectoenzymes and LTD_4-binding proteins which develop during maturation and differentiation. Furthermore, the technique of direct photoaffinity labeling with leukotrienes is useful for identifying leukotriene-binding proteins on cellular membranes.

FUSION OF MONOCYTES AND TUMOR CELLS IN VITRO

Johannes Möst, Ludwig Spötl, Manfred P. Dierich

Institut für Hygiene, Leopold-Franzens-Universität Innsbruck, Austria

Several observations suggest that fusion of tumor cells with normal monocytes or lymphocytes could be involved in the induction of tumor metastasis. However, it is not clear, how such a fusion process could be initiated in vivo. In vitro it is possible to induce fusion of monocytes, leading to the generation of multinucleated giant cells, by incubation with a supernatant of Con A-stimulated mononuclear cells. We tested if such a conditioned medium could also induce fusion between monocytes and tumor cells. Monocytes isolated from peripheral blood of healthy donors and cells of various tumor lines were membrane-labeled with two different dyes. Monocytes and tumor cells were mixed and incubated with appropriate concentrations of the conditioned medium. The formation of multinucleated giant cells was monitored with an inverted microscope equipped for dual wave-length fluorescence. For some of the tumor cell lines (e.g., U937) no evidence of fusion with monocytes was found. In other experiments (e.g., with TALL or Sk-Mel 37) giant cells stained with both fluorochromes were observed, indicating that these cells contained membranes of both cell types and thus were derived from fusion of monocytes with tumor cells. These results indicate, that it is possible to induce fusion between normal monocytes and cells of certain tumor lines under conditions that could also occur in vivo.

HUMAN MACROPHAGES IN DEFENSE AGAINST CANCER IN A scid/HUMAN MODEL.

B. Mukherji, N.G. Chakraborty, T. Okino. University of Connecticut Medical School, Farmington, CT 06030, USA.

The role of human macrophages in defense against cancer was studied, in two autologous systems, in an adoptive transfer model using scid mice bearing xenografts of the respective autologous tumor cells. Plastic adherent macrophages, derived from leucophoresed blood mononuclear cells from the respective patients, were grown in large plastic flasks in AIM V medium (GIBCO) containing 100 U/ml Interleukin-2 (for the first 3 days) and 1000 U/ml of M-CSF (Genetics Institute, Cambridge MA). scid mice (C.B-17IcrJ) were grafted subcutaneously with approximately 1-2 million tumor cells (melanoma line JH-M and the renal cancer line JR-R). Depending upon the experimental design, mice grafted with the tumor cells were infused, intravenously and/or intraperitoneally, with the autologous cultured macrophages (107-108/infusion), on day one only, on day seven only, or three times weekly.

Marked tumor regressions (partial to complete) of established tumors as well as partial to complete protection from tumor growths were seen with both single and multiple infusions of the cultured macrophages. Analyses of the mechanism of the anti-tumor effect suggested that the tumor regressions were unlikely to have occurred as a result of direct cytolytic activity of the macrophages. Instead, the mode of action appeared to have been mediated by a cytokine(s) elaborated by the macrophages, acting either directly on the tumor cells or acting by recruiting a non-T cell defense system of the animals.

ELEVATED INTERLEUKIN 8 LEVELS IN BRONCHOALVEOLAR LAVAGE FLUID OF PATIENTS WITH ACQUIRED EMPHYSEMA.

Th. Muley, M. Wiebel, G. Klitsche, V. Schulz and W. Ebert
Thoraxklinik, Amalienstr. 5, 6900 Heidelberg-Rohrbach, FRG

Cigarette smoking is known to activate alveolar macrophages (AM) which can produce a variety of cytokines. Among these mediators Interleukin 8 (IL 8) could play a role in the pathogenesis of lungs emphysema. Besides its chemotactic activity on neutrophils (PMN), IL 8 leads to the release of PMN-elastase, which is thought to be responsible for the destruction of alveolar walls found in emphysema. To prove this hypothesis, IL 8 concentrations were measured in cell-free supernatants of bronchioalveolar lavage fluids (BALF) of patients with emphysema in comparison with patients suffering from other pulmonary diseases using Quantikine IL 8 Elisa Kit (R&D Systems Inc, USA). IL 8 was found to be significantly higher in the BALF of patients with emphysema compared to those without emphysema ($p<0.0001$, Wilcoxon test). Remarkably, the lowest levels of IL 8 were assessed in patients with sarcoidosis. In the non-emphysema group the highest median values were measured in smokers ($p<0.02$ vs nonsmokers, $p<0.04$ vs ex-smokers, Wilcoxon test). Within the emphysema group the difference between smokers and ex-smokers did not reach statistical significance. It is concluded that IL 8 could play a major role in the pathogenesis of lungs emphysema presumably due to the recruitment of neutrophils and their activation within the lung tissue. It could be demonstrated that smoking is a major risk factor for acquired emphysema, although it has to be noted, that there must exist additional factors besides smoking leading to the elevated IL 8 levels in the BALF of emphysema patients.

RFLP-ANALYSIS OF THE MACROPHAGE-COLONY STIMULATING FACTOR (CSF-1) GENE IN NORMAL AND AUTOIMMUNE MICE.

Müller, M., Jarck, P., Hecht, M., Hartung, H., Paul, D., Lohmann-Matthes, M.-L. and Emmendörffer, A. Fraunhofer Institute, Dept. of Immunobiology, 3000 Hannover 61.

Investigating the reasons for an increased macrophage compartment of SLE prone mice already at an age of 4 weeks in comparison to normal mice, we and others have found elevated serum levels of CSF-1, esp. in diseased MRL-lpr and BXSB mice. One possible site for this production of CSF-1 is the kidney, where an increased amount of CSF-1 mRNA could be detected, e.g. in NZB/W mice. Since structural abnormalities of the CSF-1 gene might be responsible for the dysregulation of the CSF-1 system, we assessed the CSF-1 gene for a restriction fragment length polymorphism. Using PST 1 and BAM H1, enzymes possessing one cleavage site in the CSF-1 gene, we digested DNA from normal (BALB/c, C3H/HeN) and lupus prone mice (NZB/W, MRL-lpr, MRL-+/+ and BXSB) and performed Southern blots. The results demonstrate no differences in the RFLP analysis indicating that in SLE prone mice the CSF-1 gene itself appears to be normal. Further studies on the CSF-1 gene promotor, on the stability of the CSF-1 mRNA and the degradation of the CSF-1/ CSF-1 receptor complex will probably reveal the explanation for the increased serum levels of this growth factor in SLE prone mice.

UROKINASE/PLASMINOGEN ACTIVATOR INHIBITOR-TYPE 1 COMPLEX BINDS TO THE PURIFIED α_2-MACROGLOBULIN RECEPTOR.

Evidence that cellular degradation in monocytes of urokinase receptor-bound complex is mediated by the α_2-macroglobulin receptor.

Nykjær A[*], Jensen PH[*], Petersen CM[¤], Møller B[¤], Moestrup SK[*], Holtet TL[$], Etzerodt M[$], Thøgersen HC[$], Munch M[#], Andreasen PA[#], Gliemann J[*].
Institute of Medical Biochemistry[*], Dept. of Clinical Immunology[¤], Laboratory for Gene Expression[$], Dept. of Molecular Biology[#], University of Aarhus, DK-8000, Aarhus C, Denmark.

We and others have shown that urokinase receptor (uPAR)-bound complexes between urokinase (uPA) and plasminogen activator inhibitor type-1 (uPA/PAI-1) are readily internalized and degraded in monocytes. In contrast, uPA or its aminoterminal fragment (ATF) are poorly internalized following binding to the glycosyl-phosphatidylinositol anchored uPAR. Monocytes express the α_2-macroglobulin receptor (α_2MR, a monocyte differentiation antigen). We have recently reported (FEBS Lett. **300**, 13-17 (1992)) that T-cell derived interleukin-2 activated killer cells express uPAR, but not α_2MR, and that they do not degrade uPAR-bound uPA/PAI-1.

We now report that uPA/PAI-1, but not uPA or ATF, binds to the α-chain of purified human placental two chain α_2MR. The magnitude of binding is comparable to that of the established ligands α_2-macroglobulin/proteinase complex and the novel 40-kDa α_2M-associated protein (α_2MRAP). Binding of uPA/PAI-1 is blocked by excess natural or recombinant α_2MRAP purified from a fusion protein expressed in E. coli. Binding is 80% inhibited by tPA/PAI-1, but not tPA, and 50-80% inhibited by reactive center-cleaved PAI-1, an anti PAI-1 mAb and an anti-uPA mAb against the serine proteinase domain.

In monocytes, uPA/PAI-1 is bound to uPAR (blocked by ATF), and rα_2MRAP is bound to α_2MR (blocked by α_2M/proteinase). rα_2MRAP does not inhibit binding of uPA/PAI-1 in monocytes, confirming binding of the complex to cellular uPAR. In contrast, rα_2MRAP does inhibit specific monocyte degradation of uPA/PAI-1 by about 80%.

In conclusion, purified α_2MR binds uPA/PAI-1 complex and the PAI-1 moiety seems to contribute. The data strongly suggest that α_2MR mediates cellular internalization and degradation of uPAR-bound uPA/PAI-1.

THE INTRACELLULAR RESISTANCE OF MYCOBACTERIUM FORTUITUM TO KILLING BY MONOCYTE-DERIVED MACROPHAGES

Nziramasanga P., P.M. Shah and W. Stille
Infektiologie
Zentrum der Innere Medizin
Klinikum der J.W. Goethe Universität
Theodor-Stern Kai 7
6000 Frankfurt am Main 70

Abstract

The interaction between the atypical mycobacterial species M. fortuitum and normal unstimulated human macrophages was studied in vitro using the method of Crowle and May. Blood monocytes were isolated and cultured on tissue culture plastic surfaces for 7 days in RPMI 1640 with 10% Fetal Calf Serum. The adherent cells were observed to transform into large, irregularly shaped macrophages after 4 days in culture. The mycobacteria were added to the cells at 10 000 bacteria/ml. After 1 hour incubation, extracellular bacteria were removed by washing.

The intracellular viability of M. fortuitum was assessed as colony forming units (CFU) at 2 hour intervals. The inoculum was reduced by 35% within the first 2 hours of incubation followed by no significant killing between 2 and 4 hours, and a 12% reduction in CFU between 4 and 8 hours. An increase in CFU was observed after 8 hours of incubation, indicating intracellular growth.

Ofloxacin at 0.2xMIC had no noticeable influence on the intracellular or extracellular viability of M. fortuitum. At 0.5xMIC, intracellular M. fortuitum was less inhibited than the relevant extracellular control. A similar observation was made with 1.0xMIC indicating both resistance to phagocytic killing and drug action by M. fortuitum.

THE ROLE OF TUMOR NECROSIS FACTOR IN AN EXPERIMENTAL METASTASIS MODEL.

P. Orosz, *B. Echtenacher, and *D. N. Männel
Immunochemistry, German Cancer Research Center, Heidelberg and *Tumorimmunology, Clinic of the University, Regensburg, FRG.

The role of tumor-infiltrating macrophages and the function of tumor-stimulated monocytes for tumor growth and metastasis is not clear. Enhanced production of tumor necrosis factor (TNF) by peripheral blood monocytes as well as by tumor-infiltrating macrophages *in situ* has been documented in cancer patients and in tumor-bearing animals. Augmented TNF levels could fulfill a surveillance function protecting the host from tumor growth. On the other hand, such endogenous TNF might be harmful by modifying the metastatic potential of tumor cells due to the broad spectrum of biological activities of TNF. We, therefore, investigated the influence of endogenous and exogenous TNF on metastasis in an experimental fibrosarcoma metastasis model. $3x10^5$ CFS1 cells, methylcholanthrene-induced fibrosarcoma cells, were inoculated *i.v.* into mice and pulmonary metastases were counted on day 11. The animals received either a single *i.p.* injection of recombinant human TNF (rhTNF), recombinant mouse TNF (rmTNF), or mTNF-neutralizing monoclonal antibodies (V1q) 5 hours prior to tumor injection. Both groups of TNF pretreated animals showed significant enhancement of metastases in the lung, while neutralization of endogenous TNF led to a decrease. Dose responses of rhTNF and rmTNF demonstrated a stronger metastasis-enhancing effect by rmTNF compared to rhTNF. Treatment with rmTNF or V1q on day 5 after tumor implantation resulted in no change of the metastatic potential indicating an early effect of TNF. No direct effect of rmTNF, rhTNF or V1q on the proliferation rate of tumor cells was seen *in vitro*. Histological analysis of micrometastases in the lung on day 5 revealed more metastatic foci and metabolically more active tumor cells after rmTNF pretreatment. Experiments to analyze the mechanisms of this metastasis-enhancing effect of TNF are in progress.

EFFECT OF SOLUBLE MoIFNγ-R TREATMENT ON THE DEVELOPMENT OF SPONTANEOUS AUTOIMMUNE DISEASE IN NZB/W F1 MICE.

Ozmen, L., Ryffel, B., Fountoulakis, M., Gentz, R. and Garotta, G.
Pharmaceutical Research New Technologies. F. Hoffmann-La Roche Ltd. 4002 Basel. Switzerland.

The NZB/W F1 females that develop spontaneously a SLE-like autoimmune disease were treated for 4 months with MoIFNγ ($5x10^4$ U 3x/week), mAb anti-IFNγ (100 µg 1x/week), MoIFNγ-R (100 µg 3x/week) or placebo (0.2 ml NaCl 3x/week). Up to now, the analysis of the mortality rate shows that 57% (4/7) of mice died in the placebo treated group, 87% (7/8) died in the MoIFNγ treated group whereas no death occurred neither in the mAb anti-IFNγ nor in the MoIFNγ-R treated groups. The highest score of proteinuria was reached 11, 17 and 21 weeks after the beginning of the treatment with MoIFNγ, placebo and mAb anti-IFNγ or MoIFNγ-R, respectively. These results were further confirmed by the immunohistochemistry analysis of the kidneys that showed a lower incidence of glomerulonephritis in mice treated with MoIFNγ-R or mAb anti-IFNγ. The treatments with MoIFNγ-R or mAb anti-IFNγ significantly delayed the emergence of anti-dsDNA autoantibodies. Most of the mice treated with MoIFNγ died without having developped high titers of anti-dsDNA autoantibodies. These results confirm the accelerating role of IFNγ in this pathology and show the capacity of the MoIFNγ-R in inhibiting the disease.

MICROGLIAL CELL CLONES PRESENT ANTIGEN IN VITRO

Paola Paglia, Francesca Granucci, Linda Cairns and Paola Ricciardi - Castagnoli.
CNR, Center of Cytopharmacology, University of Milano, Milano, ITALY.

To study the functional properties of microglial cells we have generated microglial cell clones from embryonic Balb/c brain cultures (E13) by immortalization with recombinant retroviruses. In previous studies we have demonstrated that microglial clones respond to physiological signals such IFN-γ and that, like primary microglial cells, they can be induced to transcribe cytokines genes such as IL-1, IL-6 and TNF-α. In addition nitric oxide synthase activity has been demonstrated in the same clones. In this report we have analyzed the ability of these microglial clones to express MHC class II molecules and present antigen. IFN-γ acts synergistically with GM-CFS to enhance the expression of MHC class II molecules. The activated microglial cells were tested for antigen presentation of Spermwhale myoglobin to a Th_1 cell hybridoma, 13.26.8-H6.1, recognizing the 132-147 myoglobin peptide in a $H\text{-}2^d$ restricted context. Fifty thousand T cell hybrids/well were cultured with the same number of APCs using the native antigen doses indicated in figure 1. After 24 hrs 100 µl aliquots of supernatant were transferred to fresh microtiter plates together with five thousand/well IL-2 dependent HT-2 cells. ^{3}H-Thymidine incorporation of HT-2 was measured 24 hours later. As shown microglial cells were able to process and present the specific antigen upon activation with IFN-γ and GM-CSF. The ability of resident microglial cells to process and present antigens in vitro raises the question of the potential APC functions of endogenous microglial cells in vivo.

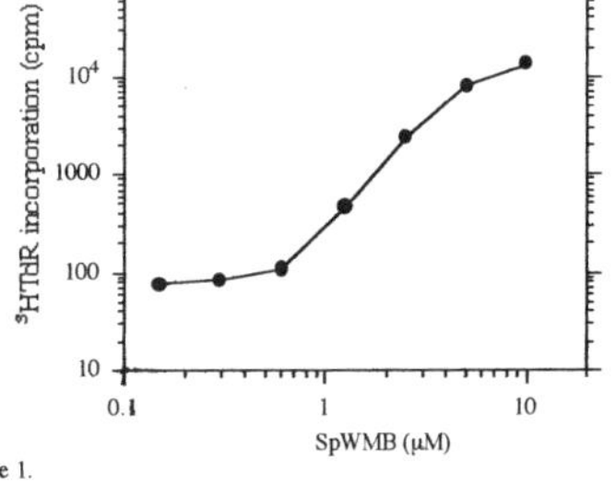

Figure 1.

MODULATION OF MONOKINE PRODUCTION BY THEMSELVES OR BY XENOBIOTICS

M.A. Parant
University Paris 6, 15 rue de l'Ecole-de-Médecine, 75270 Paris 6 France.

Circulating level of monokines following administration of a bacterial component can be modulated by various agents, including cytokines, in an intricate network. Thus, pretreatment of mice with rMuTNF or rHuTNF caused a marked enhancement in the yield of LPS-induced serum TNF, IL-1 and IL-6. In vitro and ex vivo assays have also shown the strong potentiating effect of TNF. IL-1α or β displayed differential effects. They both depressed the TNF response upon subsequent LPS challenge without affecting serum IL-6 titer, but in vitro the response of mouse macrophages to LPS (mRNA or protein) was not influenced in the presence of IL-1. Both IL-1 and IL-6 were used in assays performed in mice that had been adrenalectomized. Whereas the inhibitory effect of IL-6 on TNF production was maintained in these animals, pretreatment with IL-1 exerted a priming effect for an enhanced cytokine response to LPS. Therefore, whereas the effect of IL-6 appeared to be a direct one on TNF-producing cells, the two contradictory effects of IL-1 were indirect. The enhanced level of serum corticosterone may account for depression of TNF release in normal mice, and the stimulating effect in the absence of adrenals appeared to be related to other mediators. The potentiation of responses to LPS observed after pretreatment with muramyl dipeptides (MDP) was shown to depend on a direct action on macrophages leading to expression of mRNA of the three cytokines and to a strong increase in mRNA accumulation after the LPS challenge. The level of protein released after stimulation with MDPs was rather low in the absence of a second signal and the production of any cytokine did not seem responsible for the priming effect of the synthetic compounds.

PREVENTION OF CIRCULATORY SHOCK BY THE MONOCYTE/MACROPHAGE ACTIVATOR MTP-PE IN A PIG-MODEL OF SEPTICEMIA

Passlick,B.*, Izbicki,J.R.*, Ostertag,P. *, Löffler,Th.* and Ziegler-Heitbrock,H.W.L.°

*Dept. of Surgery and °Institute of Immunology, University of Munich, Munich, Germany

Septicemia is still a major problem in patients with polytrauma or major surgery, leading to septic shock, organ failure and death. Prevention of septic shock in patients at risk would be tempting way to face this problem. We therefore conducted a trial with the monocyte activator muramyl-tripeptide-phosphatidylethanolamine (MTP-PE) in an experimental pig model.

Material and Methods: Liposome encapsulated MTP-PE (50 µg/kg; n=5) or liposomes alone (n=5) were given i.v. 24 h before sepsis was induced by LPS (S.abortus, 4µg/kg/h). Animals were anaethesized and mechanically ventilated and monitored over an 8 h period.

Results: MTP-PE is effective in preventing LPS-induced septic shock and death: None of the MTP-PE pretreated pigs died, but 5 out of 5 control animals . The treated animals develop no fever, the arterial pressure is stable and blood oxygenation is significantlly improved. No differences between MTP-PE pretreated animals and control animals were found with respect to septic leuco- and thrombocytopenia, hemo-concentration and urinary output.

Conclusions: Monocyte activation by MTP-PE is effective in preventing septic shock and death in an experimental model.

THE CYTOSTATIC ACTIVITY ACQUIRED BY HUMAN MONOCYTES DURING THEIR DIFFERENTIATION INTO MACROPHAGES IS INDEPENDENT OF NO AND TNFα.

Jean-François Petit, Phan Bich Liên and Geneviève Lemaire, URA 1116, Bâtiment 432, Université Paris-Sud, 91405-Orsay

Chantal Martinache and Manuel Lopez, INSERM U 76, CNTS, 53 Bd Diderot, 75012-Paris.

When differentiated into macrophages in teflon bags in the presence of AB serum, human monocytes acquire a cytostatic activity against tumor cells (Andreesen et al., J. Immunol. Methods, 56, 295-304, 1983). We cultivated during seven days under these conditions either monocytes obtained by elutriation at day 0 (D_0) or mononuclear cells from which macrophages were obtained by elutriation at D_7. Cytostatic activity was monitored by coculture of D_7 macrophages and tumor cells at an effector/target ratio of 4 in the presence of tritiated thymidine.

We used two tumor cell lines insensitive to TNFα, the murine P815 mastocytoma and the human K562 erythroleukemia and one sensitive to TNFα, the U937 histiocytic lymphoma. The proliferation of the three cell lines was completely arrested in vitro by differentiated human macrophages, whether obtained from monocytes or from mononuclear cells (residual incorporation of thymidine<10%).

The macrophage cytostatic activity is not due to NO : nitrites cannot be detected in macrophage conditioned media ; the cytostatic activity is insensitive to the two classical inhibitors of NO-synthase, N-monomethyl-L-arginine and ω-nitro-L-arginine.

The cytostatic activity is also independent of TNFα. Macrophages exhibit cytostatic activity against two TNFα resistant cell lines. Moreover, even in the presence of anti-TNFα antibodies able to neutralize more than 500 U/ml TNFα, we still observed an unchanged activity against the three targets, including the U937 cell line.

We can thus conclude that human monocytes differentiated in vitro develop cytostatic mechanisms independent of NO and TNFα. Their molecular bases are currently under investigation.

HUMAN BLOOD MONOCYTES ACTIVATION BY GP 120 HIV ENVELOPE PROTEIN. EVIDENCE FOR NITRIC OXIDE RELEASE.

D. Pietraforte, E. Tritarelli*, U. Testa*, M. Minetti

Biologia Cellulare and Ematologia-Oncologia*

Istituto Superiore di Sanita', Viale Regina Elena 299, 00161 ROMA, ITALY

Purpose: Nitric oxide (NO°) was recently identified as effector of phagocytes-mediated cytostasis and/or cytotoxycity. NO°, a short-lived free radical synthesized by enzimatic oxidation of L-arginine, is an intermediate in nitrite (NO_2^-) formation. We studied the ability of HIV gp 120 protein to activate blood monocytes to produce NO° and NO_2^-.

Methods: Peripheral blood monocytes (PBM) were cultured for 0-4 days. The production of radicals was studied by spin-trapping technique. This technique involves the addition of a nitrone compound (5,5-dimethyl-1-pyrroline-N-oxide, DMPO) which is capable of rapidly trapping short-lived radicals to form more persistent nitroxide radicals (spin adducts). NO_2^- was quantified in the cell culture supernatants by using the Griess reagent.

Results and conclusions: Gp 120 at µM concentration was able to stimulate the PBM radicals production (100-200% adduct increase) and NO_2^- release (150 %). The adduct formation was not modified by superoxide dismutase, indomethacin and acetyl salicylate. An inhibition of 64 ± 7% was observed with N-nitro-L-arginine, a stereospecific inhibitor of L-arginine oxidative pathway. The hyperfine splitting constants of the adducts suggest the formation of DMPO-OH. NO° is expected to give a DMPO adduct with hyperfine splitting constants different from those observed. Nevertheless, bubbling of NO° gas in a N_2-saturated solution of DMPO gave a DMPO adduct with hyperfine splitting constants superimposable to that of DMPO-OH. The reaction leading to DMPO-OH formation from NO° is unclear.

Our data indicate that gp 120 stimulate L-arginine oxidative pathway in PBM. $NO°/NO_2^-$ release may contribute to cellular and tissutal damage of AIDS disease.

Abstract

CONCOMITTANT INCREASE OF ALVEOLAR MACROPHAGE RECEPTORS AND OF SOLUBLE RECEPTORS IN EXOGENOUS ALLERGIC ALVEOLITIS, SARCOIDOSIS AND LUNG FIBROSIS

A. Pforte[1], A. Schießler[1], S.U. Kress[1], A. Brunner[1], B. Behr[3], P. Gais[4], H.W.L. Ziegler-Heitbrock[2]

Medical Clinic, Medical Department, LMU, Munich[1]

Institute of Immunology LMU Munich[2]

Central Hospital Gauting[3]

GSF Munich[4]

All the different types of alveolitis are characterized by an increased cellularity in bronchoalveolar lavage due to an increase of T-lymphocytes and alveolar macrophages (AM). The AM are activated and we can demonstrate increased levels of IL-2R (CD25) staining in immunocytochemistry. Cytometry reveals that in allergic alveolitis 21 % of AM are IL-$2R^+$ compared to 2 % in controls. At the same time soluble serum IL-2R are increased by factor 2 with a positive correlation for IL-$2R^+$ AM and ssIL-2R. A comparable pattern is seen in sarcoidosis and in lung fibrosis. Furthermore, increased expression of CD14 in AM alveolitis patients was also associated with increased serum levels of sCD14 and ICAM-1. Response to therapy was associated with a decrease of both AM associated and soluble serum receptors. The data suggest that soluble serum receptors may be derived from AM and that serum parameters can be employed to study the status of AM in various forms of interstitial lung disease.

FUNCTIONAL AND RECEPTOR CHARACTERIZATION OF MOUSE PERITONEAL MACROPHAGES.

Nathalie Plasman and Bernard Vray.
Laboratory of Immunology, Faculty of Medicine, Free University of Brussels, 808, route de Lennik, 1070 Brussels - Belgium.

In this study, we describe, for the first time, a flow-cytometric analysis of both various membrane antigens and bacterial (opsonized or not with an immune serum) phagocytosis of mouse resident peritoneal cell fractions. The same fractions were also characterized by morphological criteria and enzymatic assays. The specific density of the cell fractions was first determined using a continuous Percoll gradient. Then, discontinuous Percoll gradients were realized in routine. This procedure improved the harvesting of all the various cell peritoneal types. The flow-cytometric analysis showed that membrane antigens detected by F4/80, M1/70 and 2.4G2 monoclonal antibodies were mostly expressed by high density macrophages. The same fractions displayed also a high rate of Fc receptor-mediated bacterial phagocytosis. Morphological criteria and enzymatic assays confirmed the appartenance of these cells to the macrophage lineage. On the whole, our results underscore that typical macrophagic antigens and bacterial phagocytosis are predominantly expressed and performed by immature macrophages. The observed differences between the mature and immature macrophage fractions could explain the functional diversity of these cells in the immune response.

TRYPANOSOMA CRUZI INFECTION OF DIFFERENT MACROPHAGE FRACTIONS ISOLATED ON PERCOLL GRADIENT.

Nathalie Plasman and Bernard Vray.
Laboratory of Immunology, Faculty of Medicine, Free University of Brussels, 808, Route de Lennik, 1070 Brussels - Belgium.

The functional heterogeneity of mouse resident peritoneal macrophages is well known. Due to this heterogeneity, one can ask if some cell fractions could be more or less sensitive to the parasite *T. cruzi*. Therefore, we have studied the *T. cruzi* infection of the 7 macrophage fractions isolated on Percoll gradient. All the cell fractions were incubated with the parasite to cell ratio of 3 to 1. After 24, 48 and 72 h of infection, the percentage of infected cells and the mean number of amastigotes per infected cells were counted. Indeed, we have observed a difference in the infection and in the multiplication of the parasite. Two cell groups were identified: - First, the mature macrophages characterized by a low infection level (especially at 72 h of infection) and - second, immature macrophages with a higher infection level. A progressive evolution in the infection level is observed from the immature to the mature fractions. These differences were also observed with the Interferon-γ activated macrophages. Immature macrophages are less permissive to the activation and more sensitive to the parasite entrance and multiplication. This could be explained by the different maturity state of the cells reflecting a functional heterogeneity already observed in our other experiments (see poster session).

ANTIGEN-PRESENTING AND ACCESSORY FUNCTION OF MONOCYTES AFTER PHAGOCYTOSIS OF BACTERIA.

J. Pryjma[1], J. Baran[1], and H.-D. Flad[2]. [1]Institute of Paediatrics, Copernicus School of Medicine, Wielicka 265, 30-663 Cracow, Poland; [2]Forschungsinstitut Borstel, D-2061 Borstel, Germany

Monocytes/macrophages (MO) are involved both in the induction and effector mechanisms of the immune response, although it is not clear whether both functions can be performed by the same cell at the same time. Therefore, we examined the antigen-presenting (APC) and accessory function (AC) of monocytes after phagocytosis of bacteria.

Peripheral blood monocytes isolated from mononuclear cells by counterflow elutriation were incubated with a suspension of bacteria (*S.aureus, E.coli, P.aeruginosa, S.enteritidis*) in the presence of fresh normal human serum under conditions where at least 80% of monocytes engulfed microorganisms. These cells were either pulsed with antigen (purified derivative of tuberculin - PPD, tetanus toxoid - TT) and used as APC for autologous T lymphocytes, or their AC function was examined in pokeweed mitogen (PWM)-activated cultures of T or T and B cells.

It has been found that phagocytosis of bacteria by MO reduces their ability to trigger antigen- and mitogen-driven proliferation. In contrast, when added to PWM-activated cultures of T and B lymphocytes, MO containing microorganisms enhanced B cell differentiation into immunoglobulin-secreting cells. The reduced proliferative response of T lymphocytes was not due to a change of the kinetics of the response or triggering of "suppressor" mechanisms. Furthermore, antigen processing was not much effected after phagocytosis of bacteria, since antigen-pulsed and paraformaldehyde-fixed cells containing bacteria were comparable to control cells as APC. In contrast as a result of phagocytosis of bacteria, a reduced expression of adhesion molecules (CD11, CD54), FcRI (CD64), CD14 and a variable reduction of HLA-DQ and HLA-DP molecules was observed. In conclusion, phagocytosis of bacteria by MO affects their APC and AC functions presumably due to changes in the expression of molecules essential for MO-T cell interactions.

(Supported by grant KBN 2040/4/91 of the Polish Research Committee)

MOLECULAR PATHOGENESIS OF MONOCYTES/MACROPHAGES HIV-1 INFECTION

H. Raoul[(1)], R. Le Naour[(1)], A. Mabondzo[(1)], F. Boussin[(1)] and D. Dormont[(1,2)].
(1). Laboratoire de Neuropathologie expérimentale et Neurovirologie, CRSSA/DSV/DPTE, CEA, Fontenay-aux-Roses, France. (2). Institut Pasteur, Paris, France.

Objectives: Because clinical and biological features indicate that a dysregulation of both cytokine pattern, and microbicidal activity occurs in the monocytes/macrophages of HIV-1 infected patients, the regulation of TNFα synthesis as well as MnSOD gene expression during macrophage HIV infection, has been investigated. As previously reported, HIV-1/LAI infected macrophages did not produce any biologically detectable TNFα within the few hours following lentiviral infection, whereas a high expression of the MnSOD and TNFα genes was observed 2 and 4 hours after the infection. In this view, we attempt to determine 1) the consequence on the regulation of TNFα synthesis as well as MnSOD gene expression using monocytotropic HIV-1 strains (HIV-1/DAS and HIV-1/PAR) 2) the infectious events involved in these phenomena, testing the effects of heat inactivated virus (LAI, DAS, PAR), and recombinant GP160 (rGP160) on the macrophages.
Methods: Human peripheral blood monocytes (PBM) were obtained from healthy HIV-1 seronegative donors using the centrifugal elutriation technique. They were cultured by adherence in RPMI 1640 supplemented with 10% fetal calf serum for 7 days for differentiation into macrophages. Cells were then infected with HIV-1/DAS or HIV-1/PAR (0,001 TCID50/cell), or treated with heat inactivated HIV-1 strains (56°C, 30 mn) or rGP160 (10ng/10^6cells). Culture supernatants were harvested every 2 hours during the first 10 hours, for a TNFα biological activity test using Actinomycine D-treated L-929 cells. Concomitantly, expression levels of the MnSOD and TNFα genes were determined by Northern blots analysis.
Results: Contrarily to the results obtained with HIV-1/LAI, biological active TNFα was detectable during the early phase of *in vitro* infection of human macrophage cultures with the 2 monocytotropic strains tested. The results were the same when the different HIV-1 strains used were inactivated. No TNFα release was detectable in the supernatants of macrophage rGP160 stimulated. At the molecular level, between 2 and 4 hours after infection, an increase of TNFα and MnSOD mRNA levels was observed compared to negative control, the virus being either inactivated or not. While these expressions decreased after 4 hours, and reached control values 10 hours p.i.with HIV-1/LAI, no decrease was observed until 10 hours using HIV-1/DAS and PAR strains. Treatment with rGP160 does not change the expression level of these 2 genes in the macrophages compared to control cultures.
Conclusion: The detection of biologically active TNFα and the increase of TNFα and MnSOD gene expression in the macrophage cultures is apparently related to the cellular tropism of the viral strains used. These results may reflect an enhancement of the infection. The results obtained with all the inactivated viral strains indicate that the phenomena observed are related to the viral entry. Therefore, the binding of the rGP160 does not seems to be sufficient to induce TNFα or MnSOD expression. Experiments to test the viral specificity and to assess the mechanisms involved in the macrophagic response observed are now in progress, and results will be presented during the meeting.

THE TOXICITY OF OXIDIZED LOW DENSITY LIPOPROTEIN TOWARDS MACROPHAGES *IN VITRO*

Reid, V.C., Mitchinson, M.J.

Department of Pathology, Division of Genetic and Cellular Pathology, University of Cambridge, CB2 1QP, England.

The characteristic lipid-laden foam cells that predominate in the intima in the early stages of human atherosclerosis are known to be macrophages. The more advanced lesions have a necrotic centre, and this appears to be due principally to macrophage necrosis.

There is now considerable evidence that lipoprotein oxidation occurs within the developing atherosclerotic lesion. Macrophages can oxidize low density lipoprotein (LDL) *in vitro*. The properties of oxidized LDL have aroused a lot of interest in the study of atherosclerosis. One property which is of particular interest is its toxicity towards various cell types found in the atherosclerotic lesion in the artery wall. These have included endothelial cells and smooth muscle cells.

Since, however, it appears that the necrosis in the advanced stages of the disease is due to macrophages dying we decided to investigate whether macrophage-mediated lipoprotein oxidation was toxic for the macrophages. We looked at artificial lipoprotein preparations containing the main cholesteryl esters found within LDL and known to be oxidized *in vivo*. We also looked at oxidized LDL itself. Both were toxic to mouse peritoneal macrophages *in vitro* and this toxicity was reduced by the addition of antioxidant. The results might explain the important event of the onset of necrosis in the developing human lesion.

PROSTAGLANDIN AND LEUKOTRIENE SYNTHESIS IN A MACROPHAGE HYBRID CELL LINE (H4-7)

J. Riese and V. Kaever

Institute of Molecular Pharmacology, Medical School, D-3000 Hannover 61, FRG

Studies on the regulation of macrophage eicosanoid synthesis are often hampered by the inability of most macrophage-like cell lines to secrete measurable amounts of arachidonate 5-lipoxigenase (5-LX) products. In contrast to the commonly used cell lines RAW264.7, PU5-1.8, or P388D_1 the newly established mouse macrophage hybrid cell line H4-7 [1] was able to produce prostaglandins (PG) as well as leukotrienes (LT) upon calcium ionophore stimulation.

As shown by Western blotting (specific antisera were kindly provided by Merck Frosst, Canada) H4-7 cells contain 5-LX and 5-LX activating protein (FLAP). Addition of ionomycin to intact H4-7 cells led to a concentration- (optimum at 2.5 µg/ml) and time- (maximal after 5 min) dependent translocation and activation of 5-LX and subsequent LTC_4 synthesis (determined by ELISA). LTC_4 production was inhibited by the specific 5-LX translocation inhibitor MK886 (Merck Frosst, Canada).

We have used H4-7 cells as model system for macrophage in vitro activation. Addition of lipopolysaccharide (from Salmonella abortus equi) and recombinant murine $interferon_{gamma}$ led to an enhancement of nitric oxide (measured as NO_2^- by Griess reagent) and tumor necrosis factor (measured by bioassay) synthesis. In this in vitro system we are currently investigating changes in PG and LT production during macrophage activation.

1 Higuchi M, Higashi N, Taki H, Osawa T: J Immunol 1990; 144: 1425-1432

MACROPHAGE ACTIVATION BY MYCOPLASMA ARTHRITIDIS-DERIVED SUPERANTIGEN (MAS) NEEDS MORE THAN I-Eα OF MOUSE MHC-CLASS II

L. Rink[1], W. Nicklas[2], M. Koester[1], M. Reuter[1] and H. Kirchner[1]

[1]Institute of Immunology and Transfusion Medicine, University of Lübeck, Medical School, Lübeck, FRG, and [2]German Cancer Research Center, Heidelberg, FRG

Mycoplasma arthritidis produces a potent T cell mitogen, which belongs to the previously described group of superantigens. Mycoplasma arthritidis-derived superantigen (MAS) has a specificity for distinct Vβ-regions of the T cell receptor (TCR) like every superantigen. In contrast to other superantigens MAS also has a specificity for the MHC class-II subtype and appears to be capable of activating monocytes even in the absence of T cells. Only murine cells expressing an intact I-Eα molecule respond to MAS. In this study we show that not all I-Eα positive cells respond to MAS. Raw 264.7 and J 774.2 murine monocytic cell lines respond to MAS as do murine bone marrow-derived macrophages. Responses were measured by IL-1 and TNF-α production. On the other hand P 388 d1, Wehi 3b and M 1 murine monocytic cell lines were not stimulated by MAS. All of these cell lines were definitely I-Eα positive and able to produce IL-1 and TNF-α after induction with other stimulants. It was shown by other investigators that I-Eα transfected fibroblasts respond to MAS. However, the L 929 murine fibroblast cell line which was strongly I-Eα positive after treatment with IFN-γ did not react to MAS stimulation. From these data, we conclude that there must be a receptor for MAS, different from I-Eα. Maybe for this reason MAS, in contrast to other superantigens, directly activates monocytes.

THE UPTAKE OF *BORRELIA BURGDORFERI*: A PROMISING MODEL FOR MEMBRANE PROCESSING DURING PHAGOCYTOSIS

MG RITTIG[a], T HÄUPL[b], UE SCHAIBLE[c], M MODOLLEL[c], MM SIMON[c], GR BURMESTER[b]

From the [a]Department of Anatomy I and the [b]Institute of Clinical Immunology and Rheumatology, Department of Medicine III, University of Erlangen-Nürnberg, Erlangen, Germany, and the [c]Max-Planck-Institut für Immunbiologie, Freiburg, Germany.

We performed an electron microscopal study on the uptake of the spirochete *Borrelia burgdorferi* by human and murine phagocytes from different lineages. The spirochetes have a diameter of 0.25 µm but a length of up to 30 µm. As a consequence, these organisms are at least twice as long as most phagocytes. The uptake of such material may present a particular problem. - Our study revealed that the spirochetes were preferentially internalized via coiling phagocytosis. A sheath-like cell protrusion wrapped around a part of a spirochete in multiple turns. This led to a cylindrical coil-like complex which subsequently was internalized. The clefts between the pseudopod rotations were continuous with the extracellular space until the adjacent membranes of the coiled pseudopod fused and dissolved. In contrast, in conventional phagocytosis a part of a spirochete was dragged into the phagocyte where vacuoles developed along its line. The clefts between the invaginated cell membranes also were continuous with the extracellular space until the membrane fusion. - Ultrastructural studies have shown that intermediate stages in endosome formation are connected to the cell surface via narrow necks. Regarding the uptake of *B. burgdorferi* cells, invaginations stretched along the entire length of the spirochete sections internalized. These clefts were occupying a considerable area of the cell membrane. Due to the multiple wrapping, these membrane areas were more extensive during coiling phagocytosis as compared to conventional phagocytosis. - In summary, membrane events which are not usually encountered during the uptake of other material are displayed to a large extent during the phagocytosis of *B. burgdorferi*. In addition, other unusual features are regularly observed which have been only reported as occasional events so far. The phagocytosis of *B. burgdorferi* may serve as a promising model for membrane processing during phagocytosis.

DIFFERENTIAL INDUCTION OF MACROPHAGE EARLY GENES, c-fos, KC, JE AND TNF-ALPHA BY LIPOARABINOMANNAN FROM VIRULENT AND AVIRULENT STRAINS OF MYCOBACTERIUM TUBERCULOSIS

Roach TIA, Chatterjee D, Blackwell JM; Dept. Medicine, University of Cambridge, Addenbrooke's Hospital, England

Lipoarabinomannan (LAM) is a major cell-wall associated glycolipid produced by Mycobacterium tuberculosis and Mycobacterium leprae. The purification of LAM from the avirulent H37Ra strain and the virulent Erdman strain of M. tuberculosis revealed that these molecules differed in the structures at their non-reducing termini. The ability of the H37Ra LAM compared with the Erdman LAM to activate murine bone marrow-derived macrophages, in terms of inducing the expression of the immediate early genes c-fos, KC, JE and TNF-α, in the absence or presence of IFN-γ has been investigated. H37Ra LAM stimulated macrophage expression of c-fos, KC and JE mRNA at 100ng/ml, and TNF-α was measured in the supernatants of macrophages stimulated with 100-1000ng/ml of H37Ra LAM. By contrast, Erdman LAM was unable to induce the expression of any of the early genes in doses up to 1000ng/ml. IFN-γ (25U/ml) alone was a potent stimulus of JE mRNA expression, dominating any response obtained using IFN-γ and either H37Ra or Erdman LAM simultaneously. However, IFNγ inhibited H37Ra stimulation of KC expression. Stimulation of the macrophages with H37Ra LAM and IFN-γ resulted in enhanced levels of TNF-α production compared with those induced by H37Ra LAM alone, and macrophage supernatants also contained increased levels of nitrite. The phenomenon of avoiding the stimulation of an initial macrophage response in terms of the induction of immediate early gene expression may be an important factor in the determination of mycobacterial virulence.

INTERFERON INDUCTION BY HIV-INFECTED MONOCYTES/MACROPHAGES.

K. Rokos and G. Pauli, AIDS-Zentrum des Bundesgesundheitsamtes, Robert Koch-Institut, Nordufer 20, D-1000 Berlin 65, Germany.

Increasing evidence points to a crucial role of cells of the monocyte/macrophage (MDM) lineage in the pathogenesis and progression of HIV-infection. The dysregulation of normal cell differentiation of MDM, mediated by cytokines, may be involved in the persistence of HIV. Interferons (IFNs) seem to be important in this respect as they participate in the defence against viral and non-viral infectious pathogens. IFN-alpha as well as IFN-gamma are detected in sera of HIV-infected patients. However, HIV-infected MDM do not produce IFN; peripheral blood lymphocytes (PBL) of HIV-infected patients have a reduced capacity to produce IFN in vitro. We could show the induction of high titers of IFN activity by HIV-infected MDM upon cell-cell interaction with PBL. MDM from healthy donors, infected with HIV-1 strain HTLV-IIIB, were cocultured with PBL of healthy donors at day 8-10 p.i. at a ratio of 1:5 to 1:10. IFN activity in supernatants was determined by bioassay (WISH cells, VSV) and viral replication by HIV-1 p24. IFN titers increased up to several thousand U/ml depending upon HIV replication during 24-48 hours. Mock-infected MDM did not induce IFN activity. IFNs were composed of IFN-alpha and IFN-gamma as shown by neutralisation by specific antisera; the results point to strong synergy of both IFNs. GM-CSF treatment of MDM increased IFN production. Activation of MDM by HIV-induced IFNs was indicated by neopterin release. HIV-induced IFNs showed anti-HIV activity comparable to recombinant IFN-alpha. HIV-induced IFN production could be increased by priming of MDM with IFN-gamma prior to cocultivation with PBL.

IFN induction by HIV-infected MDM through cell-cell interaction with lymphocytes differs from the classical pathway, where the virus-infected cells themselves produce IFN. IFN induction by HIV-infected MDM points to production of endogenous host resistance factors which, through their dual antiviral and immune modulating properties, may influence natural history and course of HIV infection.

ABNORMAL INTERACTION OF MONONUCLEAR PHAGOCYTES WITH LIPOPROTEINS IN TANGIER DISEASE

G. Rothe, E. Kovacs, G. Schmitz
Institute for Clinical Chemistry, University of Regensburg, Regensburg, F.R.G.

Tangier disease is a rare autosomal recessive disorder characterized by the absence of normal high density lipid lipoproteins (HDL) in plasma and cholesteryl ester deposition in the spleen and reticuloendothelial system (RES). Previous studies suggested that an impaired cellular metabolism of HDL is the cause of plasma HDL deficiency. The mechanism of the selective cholesteryl ester deposition and macrophage accumulation in the RES but not in the vessel wall such as in atherosclerosis is, however, far less clear. Therefore the goal of the present study was the flow cytometric characterization of peripheral blood monocyte function and differentiation in blood samples from Tangier patients. Tangier monocytes freshly drawn from peripheral blood did not differ from normal monocytes in their oxidative burst response to phorbol myristate acetate, Na^+/H^+-antiport dependent alkalinization upon TNF-α exposure, or lysosomal cysteine proteinase activity. They, however, showed a significant reduction of the differentiation and activation markers CD14, HLA-DR, and CD25 when compared to normal monocytes. When monocytes isolated by monocytapheresis and countercentrifugal elutriation were cultured for 1 day in the presence of lipoproteins, Tangier monocytes in addition showed only a low activation by HDL_3 and an impaired response to TNF-α suggesting an abnormal signal transduction in these cells. High level expression of the adhesion molecules CD11b, CD44, CD48, and CD58 and the membrane bound complement regulatory proteins CD11b, CD18, CD46 and CD59 was induced following 7 day maturation of Tangier monocytes into a macrophage-like morphology in the presence of HDL_2, HDL_3, or oxidized LDL. These results suggest that splenomegaly and macrophage accumulation in the RES of Tangier patients are associated with a defect in cellular signal transduction in response to HDL interaction. This may be both related to the primary genetic defect in the intracellular processing of HDL and to the selective depletion of mature monocytes. A further characterization of monocyte function in Tangier patients should be helpful for understanding the role of mononuclear phagocytes in atherogenesis.

INDUCING DIFFERENTIATION OF DENDRITIC CELLS FROM HUMAN BLOOD MONOCYTES *IN VITRO*

J. Ruppert[1,2], H. Xu[1], R.K.H. Gieseler[1], U. Friedrichs[1], H.P. Spengler[1], C. Schütt[3] and J.H. Peters[1]

[1]Dep. of Immunology, Georg-August-University, Göttingen, FRG; [2]Cytel Corp., San Diego, CA, U.S.A.; [3]Dep. Medical Immunology, Ernst-Moritz-Arndt-University, Greifswald, FRG.

Under serum containing culture conditions human peripheral blood monocytes (Mo) differentiate into mature macrophages (Mph) *in vitro*. Alternatively, under serum-free conditions Mo can differentiate into highly accessory cells which exhibit dendritic cell (DC) function and phenotype.

IL-4 (30 U/ml) was found to downregulate expression of CD14, a key marker distinguishing Mo/Mph from DC. This downregulation was supported by an attachment-free isolation and cultivation of Mo on agarose (2%). However, IL-4 (20 U/ml) failed to downregulate CD14 when Mo were cultured on tissue culture plastic without serum. GM-CSF (100 U/ml) was found to be able to replace serum in supporting the regulatory effect of IL-4 on CD14 expression. The downregulation of CD14 expression results from shedding of CD14 molecules as well as suppression of CD14 mRNA transcription. Moreover, the IL-4 treatment increased Mo accessory activity when they were used as stimulator cells of an allogeneic mixed lymhpocyte reaction. GM-CSF synergized the effect of IL-4 in the upregulation of Mo accessory activity.

In conclusion, Mo cultered under certain conditions exhibit a dendritic cell-like phenotype, and a high accessory activity comparable to that of DC. This supports our hypothesis that DC may originate from Mo.

ZYMOSAN-INDUCED TYROSINE PHOSPHORYLATIONS IN HUMAN MONOCYTES: ROLE OF PROTEIN KINASE C

Muriel-Véronique Sanguedolce*, Christian Capo*, Mohamad Bouhamdan*, Pierre Bongrand*, Chi-Kuang Huang#, Jean-Louis Mege*.

*Laboratoire d'Immunologie, Hôpital de Sainte-Marguerite, 270 Bd de Sainte-Marguerite, 13009 Marseille, France.#Department of Pathology, University of Connecticut, Health Center, Farmington, CT 06032, USA.

Protein tyrosine phosphorylations are involved in the proliferation and secretory responses of immune cells but their role in phagocytes is poorly understood. The ability of unopsonized zymosan to induce protein tyrosine phosphorylations was investigated in human monocytes. The addition of zymosan to monocytes resulted in an increase in tyrosine phosphorylation of several endogenous proteins. 55 and 62 kD proteins were the predominant phosphoproteins and their level of phosphorylation was rapidly increased. 38, 42, 47, 68, 90, 110, 116 and 120 kD proteins were phosphorylated with a delayed kinetics. As zymosan binds mainly to CR3 receptor on human monocytes and as CR3 is devoid of intrinsic tyrosine kinase activity, it is predictable that zymosan stimulated a tyrosine kinase distal to the receptor. We observed that phorbol myristate acetate mimicked zymosan-induced tyrosine phosphorylations, thus suggesting that both agonists used a common transductional pathway implicating the serine/threonine kinase, protein kinase C. The antagonists of protein kinase C, sphingosine and calphostin C, inhibited zymosan-stimulated tyrosine phosphorylations. We suggest that, in human monocytes, zymosan-induced tyrosine phosphorylations require the sequential activation of protein kinase C and cellular protein tyrosine kinases.

ACTIVATION OF MONONUCLEAR PHAGOCYTES BY IMMUNOTHERAPY WITH HIGH DOSE IL-2 - COMPARISON WITH AN IFNγ PROTOCOL

Carmen Scheibenbogen, Ulrich Keilholz, Werner Hunstein. Med. Poliklinik, Hospitalstr. 3, 6900 Heidelberg, FRG.

The rationale of IL-2-based immunotherapy is the activation of T lymphocytes and NK cells, whereas the classical compound to stimulate macrophage cytotoxicity is IFNγ. Monocytes and macrophages, however, also express the intermediate affinity chain of the IL-2 receptor (p75), and it has been shown in vitro that IL-2 can stimulate monocyte cytotoxicity.
We therefore studied the effect of high dose IL-2 infusion on mononuclear phagocytes in vivo. High dose IL-2 infusion results in plasma levels sufficient to saturate the median affinity chain of the IL-2 receptor. To monitor the activation of mononuclear phagocytes, neopterin, which is only released by these cells upon several stimuli, is a very useful marker. Neopterin serum levels increased 18 hours after starting the IL-2 infusion and steadily rose until the last day of therapy. Maximal levels of neopterin were 44.5±6.6 nmol/l (SEM, n=10), pretreatment levels were 8.5+2.4 nmol/l (SEM, n=10). A single injection of 3x10^6 units of IFNg s.c., which is considered to be the optimal dose for in vivo activation of mononuclear phagocytes, leads to maximal neopterin levels of only 17.0±2.3 nmol/l (n=7/pretreatment values 9.3±1 nmol/l).

In vitro stimulation of monocytes and macrophages with IL-2 alone could not induce neopterin. IL-2, however, was synergistic with IFNγ in stimulating neopterin release. This synergism is of relevance in high-dose IL-2 therapy since significant endogenous production of IFNγ can be detected with a maximal peak of 1.7±0.35 U/ml after 18 hours. Monocytes and macrophages activated by IFNγ and IL-2 produced high amounts of TNFα as well, while each stimulus alone could not stimulate TNFα release. This synergism can also explain the induction of high levels of TNFα observed during IL-2 therapy, but not following IFNγ therapy.

Our data provide evidence that immunotherapy with high dose IL-2 very efficiently activates mononuclear phagocytes and IFNγ and IL-2 act synergistically.

COMPARATIVE ANALYSIS OF TRANSCRIPTION AND PROTEIN RELEASE OF THE INFLAMMATORY CYTOKINES INTERLEUKIN-1 BETA (IL-1ß) AND IL-8 FOLLOWING MAJOR HUMAN TRAUMA.

C.Schinkel*, S.Zimmer*, J-P.Kremer°, A.Walz#, C.Rordorf+, S.Alkan+, E.Faist*

* University of Munich, Klinikum Großhadern, Dept. of Surgery, Munich, Germany; ° GSF Insitut for Experimental Hematology, Munich, Germany; # University of Bern, Theodor-Kocher Institut, Bern, Switzerland; + Ciba-Geigy LTD Research Laboratories, Pharmaceutical Division, Basel, Switzerland

The precondition for the systematic modulation of host impairing behaviour of hyperactivated monocytes (MØ) following trauma is to fully understand the mechanistic basis of cellular dysfunction. It was the objective of the study to scrutinize the synthesis patterns and the level of regulation of the functionally related inflammatory cytokines IL-1ß and IL-8 under stressful conditions. We were comparing the quantity of cytokine protein release in LPS (1µg/ml) stimulated in-vitro cultures of peripheral blood mononuclear leukocytes (PBMC) with the signal intensity of the corresponding mRNA´s detectable. 14 patients with major burn or multiple trauma (AVG ISS 34±8pts) and 14 healthy volunteers on consecutive days (D1,3,5,7,10) post trauma were studied. Protein release was measured via RIA (IL-1ß) respectively neutrophil-glucoronidase release bioassay (IL-8), mRNA expression following cytolysis was determined over northern blotting and radioactive hybridisation with the ^{32}P-labeled corresponding cDNA´s. The results for the calculation of the protein production of the individual MØ, expressed as synthesis factor (fIL-1ß, fIL-8), are depicted in the table (X±SEM, * $p<0.05$ vs control (C)).

	D1	D3	D5	D7	D10	C
fIL-1	3.4*±0.7	3.8±0.9	2.6*±0.7	6.6±2.4	8.8±2.2	5.5±0.8
fIL-8	114*±27	146±29	110*±27	240±52	238±80	205±33

We saw an almost identical pattern of synthesis for both monokines during the time of observation, with a considerable impairment until D5 and recovery thereafter. While for IL-8 in the majority of patients a clear concurrence between the mRNA signal intensity and the quantity of protein release was found, only in 3 out of 14 patients this was also the case for IL-1ß. From these data we conclude that the launching mechanisms for the de-novo synthesis for both monokines under stress differ greatly, with IL-8 being clearly regulated on the transcriptional level, while the downregulation of IL-1ß, initially post trauma, occurs most likely on the posttranscriptional level.

SYNERGISTIC INHIBITION OF THE RELEASE OF REACTIVE NITROGEN INTERMEDIATES FROM MURINE MACROPHAGES BY INTERLEUKIN-4 AND TRANSFORMING GROWTH FACTOR-BETA OR 2,4-DIAMINO,6-HYDROXY-PYRIMIDINE AND DEXAMETHASONE

Markus Schneemann, Gabriele Schoedon, Lourdes Guerrero, Gian Flury and Andreas Schaffner

Department of Medicine, University Hospital, CH-8091 Zürich, Switzerland

Reactive nitrogen intermediates (RNI) are proposed to belong to non-oxidative killing mechanisms in mononuclear phagocytes and to mediate vasodilatation, for example in endotoxin shock. Important amounts of RNI are secreted by resident and inflammatory murine macrophages after induction of NO-synthase (NOS) in vitro. Most powerful inductors are LPS, IFN-γ and the combination thereof. Induction of NOS can be counteracted by different cytokines and some pharmacological agents: a) IL-4 and TGF-β dramatically inhibit release of RNI by LPS and IFN-γ-stimulated murine peritoneal macrophages. b) Dexamethasone directly suppresses induction of NOS by LPS and IFN-γ and synergizes with c) 2,4-diamino,6-hydroxypyrimidine (DAHP), an inhibitor of de novo-biosynthesis of tetrahydrobiopterin (BH4), an obligate cofactor of NOS. d) DAHP itself appears to inhibit NOS, since release of RNI cannot be completely restored by sepiapterin, an analogue of BH4. Accordingly, inhibition of NOS by DAHP protects mice in vivo from lethal endotoxin shock ($P < 0.05$). We conclude that NOS is an important target for regulation by biological immunomodulators (LPS, IFN-γ, IL-4, TGF-β) as well as by glucocorticoids or antagonist of cofactor-biosynthesis which might be exploited for treatment of experimental endotoxin shock.

THE ROLE OF MONONUCLEAR PHAGOCYTES IN THE PATHOGENESIS OF ATHEROSCLEROSIS

G. Schmitz, E. Kovacs, G. Rothe
Institute for Clinical Chemistry and Laboratory Medicine, University of Regensburg

In atherosclerosis mononuclear phagocytes play a key role in the destruction of the vessel wall through endothelial adherence and invasion of circulating monocytes, induction of smooth muscle cell proliferation through the secretion of growth factors, and transformation into lipid-loaded foam cells or activated cells. It is not clear, however, whether phenotypic or functional alterations of peripherally circulating monocytes and their subpopulations may be an independent factor in the pathogenesis of atherosclerosis as suggested by the occurrence of atherosclerosis in only a subset of patients with hypercholesterolemia and in contrast macrophage accumulation in the spleen and RES in the genetic plasma HDL deficiency of Tangier disease. Therefore, in this study the expression of activation and differentiation markers (CD14, CD16, CD4, CD64, HLA-DR), membrane bound complement regulatory proteins (CD11b, CD18, CD25, CD35, CD46, CD55, CD59) and adhesion molecules (CD11a, CD48, CD58) was studied on monocytes from freshly drawn blood of patients with hypercholesterolemia and Tangier disease. The hypercholesterolemic patients were divided into two groups according to the presence (CHD^+) or lack of (CHD^-) coronary heart disease. A significant decrease of differentiation, activation markers and membrane bound complement components was detectable on monocytes from CHD^+ and Tangier patients suggesting either a downregulation of surface receptors or the selective depletion of mature monocytes. This hypothesis was further supported by the reduction of the $CD14^+/CD16^+$ subpopulation in CHD^+ patients. To study the effects of lipoproteins on circulating monocytes, mononuclear phagocytes from healthy controls and a Tangier patient were cultured for 1-7 days in the presence of LDL, its modified forms (acLDL, oxLDL), HDL_2 and HDL_3. LDL and its modified forms as well as HDL subclasses induced higher expression of the complement regulatory proteins and adhesion molecules during the culture of monocytes from controls. In Tangier disease in contrast the markers were down regulated by HDL subclasses. A reduced oxidative burst was furthermore detected in 1 day HDL_3 cultured Tangier monocytes. In prolonged culture of 7 days, monocytes showed a retarded expression of HLA-DR, CD14 and CD4 in the presence of the LDL derived fractions, but an increase of the $CD14^+/CD16^+$ subpopulation in the case of HDL subfractions in controls. In contrast, 7 day cultured Tangier monocytes reacted with an enormous expression of complement regulatory proteins and adhesion molecules in the case of HDL_2, HDL_3 and oxLDL suggesting an altered signal transduction of monocytes in Tangier disease. On the basis of our results we conclude that the heterogeneity and priming of circulating monocytes is an independent indicator for the atherogenic risk during hypercholesterolemia or splenomegaly in Tangier disease and should be of value for the development and evaluation of new therapeutical approaches.

NATURAL SOLUBLE HUMAN CD14 (sCD14) PREVENTS BINDING OF LPS TO MONOCYTES AND THEIR ACTIVATION

C. Schütt, C. Krüger, T. Schilling, U. Grunwald.
Dept. Med. Immunology, Ernst-Moritz-Arndt-University, Greifswald, Germany.

Binding of the LPS:LBP complex to monocytes via CD14 causes them to be activated and release large amounts of cytotoxic factors including TNF or oxygen radicals. This activation is thought to be the major pathway leading to endotoxin shock; therefore inhibition of cell activation might provide an useful theory. Purified native, spontaneous released soluble CD14 is a functionally active receptor. The specifity of endotoxin binding by sCD14 could be demonstrated using blocking and non blocking anti CD14 antibodies. sCD14 inhibits the binding of FITC-LPS to both human and bovine monocytes. In comparison to human CD14 the binding affinity of bovine CD14 to LBP-LPS-complexes is lower. Human CD14 suppresses the LPS-inducible oxidative burst response of normal monocytes. Its suppressive capacity works even in the case of CD14-negative monocytes of PNH patients which were highly responsible to LPS activation in vitro. The potential of sCD14 as a new therapeutic for septic shock is being evaluated.

THE RELEVANCE OF SUPPORTING AND NEUTRALIZING COMPOUNDS IN BODY FLUIDS FOR CELLULAR ACTIVATION BY ENDOTOXINS

C. Schütt, C. Krüger, F. Stelter, T. Schilling, S. Witt, K. Vaczi, U. Grunwald
Dept. Med. Immunology, Ernst-Moritz-Arndt-University, Greifswald, Germany

The measurement of endotoxin concentrations in patients blood is not of prognostic relevance for their outcome. However, serum proteins like HDL, LPS-binding proteins (LBP, Septin) or sCD14 can influence the cellular activation via CD14 or other receptors and its further consequences. The binding of LPS to CD14 is mediated by purified LBP, this function of LBP is not species restricted. There seems to be a different affinity of CD14 to endotoxins in different species as well as between membrane bound and soluble CD14 in the human system. The soluble form is functionally active. It seems likely that the relationship between LBP and sCD14 in different species reflects their different endotoxin sensitivity. Endotoxins and different cytokines regulate the production of sCD14 and LBP. Soluble CD14 is able to interfere with activation of CD14-negative cells by LPS too. Using a lot of anti CD14mAb we could demonstrate, that there is a variation in epitope expression on human CD14 during monocyte/macrophage differentiation or granulocyte activation which raised many new questions. These results indicate, that a multiparameter monitoring looking for HDL-, LBP-, and sCD14-concentrations can realize a more detailed view of patients situation.

INFLUENCE OF PAF AND LTB_4 ON THE RELEASE OF CYTOKINES AND SUPEROXIDE ANION BY DIFFERENTIATED HL-60-CELLS AND ALVEOLAR MACROPHAGES

I. Lind, A. Seidel
Kernforschungszentrum Karlsruhe, Institut für Genetik und Toxikologie, Postfach 3640, D-7500 Karlsruhe 1, Germany

In experimental toxicology one single cell type is usually exposed in vitro to the noxious agent and then, for example, the release of cytokines or superoxide anion is measusred. In vivo granulocytes and macrophages may be subject to the influence of lipid mediators which are released by other components of the tissue and which could possibly modulate the response of the test cells. The aim of our study was to determine whether potent lipid mediators such as PAF or LTB_4 could induce the production of some cytokines and superoxide by themselves and whether they can modulate the stimulus (LPS- or Zymosan) induced release of these mediators.

HL-60 cells were differentiated to granulocytes (HL-60-G) by 1.3% DMSO or macrophages (HL-60-M) by Calcitriol (10^{-6}M) and cultivated on membranes directly in gas phase. It was found that the cells can secrete the cytokines into the culture medium below the membranes. LPS (10 µg/ml) is a potent inducer for the release of TNF, IL-6 and IL-8 by HL-60-G as well as HL-60-M. PAF alone (1 ng/ml) does not cause any secretion of these cytokines. It has no effect at all on the response of both cell types towards LPS stimulation. Bovine alveolar macrophages (BAM) obtained by post-mortem lavage were also kept in gas phase. In this case, the secretion of a TNF-like activity had to be determined by the cytotoxicity of the medium to WEHI cells. As with HL-60 cells, BAM secrete TNF when stimulated with LPS. Neither PAF nor LTB_4 (20 nM) showed any effect when applied as single substance. In analogy to the findings reported above, their combination with LPS did not change the stimulus-induced TNF production. PAF was also not able to stimulate any superoxide anion release, neither in gas phase culture nor in normal culture conditions.

Summing up, the results suggest that PAF seems not to play an important role in the regulation of the response of macrophages and granulocytes to stimuli. By itself it has no influence on the release of some important proinflammatory mediators by macrophages and granulocytes.

ACCESSORY CELLS DERIVED FROM MONOCYTES RESEMBLE LANGERHANS CELLS IN PHENOTYPE AND PRIMARY MLR

Falko Steinbach and Bernhard Thiele*
Institut für Virologie, FU Berlin and *Charité, HU Berlin

It has been shown earlier that human peripheral blood monocytes can be differentiatiated into accessory cells (1) and that an alternative way of differentiation leads to a Langerhans cell phenotype, which we lately described first (2).

For this purpose, we isolated monocytes via Ficoll-paque and selective adherence to plastic dishes. As shown by Giemsa-staining and trypan blue exclusion, the obtained purity is >95% and viability >98%. Functional activity has been measured by non-specific esterase and phagocytosis of Candida albicans. Surface markers were investigated using flow cytometry.

The analysis of surface markers characterizes the cells as $CD1^+$ and CD14 $^+$ or $^-$, depending on the stage of differentiation. As CD1 is an originally lymphocyte marker, and CD14 picks only a subpopulation of these cells, we tried to define further criteria for morphological characterization of monocytic accessory cells. As a result, we provide evidence that, by using mannosyl-BSA-FITC, lectins like the mannose-receptor are highly sufficient homogenous markers for all populations of monocytic cells.

Dense cultures of human peripheral blood monocytes often show a proliferative activity, but it has to be underlined that proliferation is not required for the generation of this phenotype. Our recent studies on the lymphocyte stimulating capacity in a mixed lymphocyte reaction have further demonstrated that the monocyte-derived cells resemble Langerhans cells in phenotype function.

1) H.M. Najar, A.C. Bru-Capdeville, R.K.H. Gieseler and J.H. Peters, *Eur. J.Cell Biol.*,51:339 (1990)
2) Rossi,Hevcker,Gelderblom,Thiele and Steinbach, *Imm. Lett.*, 31, 189-98 1992

PYRROLIDINE-DITHIOCARBAMATE (PDTC) INHIBITS BOTH NFκB MOBILIZATION AND TNF PRODUCTION IN HUMAN MONOCYTES.

T.Sternsdorf, M. Ströbel, A. Wedel, R. Schreck, P.A. Bäuerle, H.W.L. Ziegler-Heitbrock. Institute for Immunology, University of Munich, MPI for Biochemistry, Martinsried

Lipopolysaccharide (LPS) stimulation of human Mono Mac 6 cells will result in a rapid and transient transcription of the TNF gene with a maximum at 2 hs. Preceeding this transcriptional activation there is a mobilization of the nuclear factor NFκB as detected by binding of a p50 homodimer and a p50/p65 heterotetramer to a -605 motif in the TNF promoter. In order to demonstrate that the transcriptional activation is mediated by NFκB, we have blocked NFκB mobilization with PDTC (300 µM at -1 h). Such treatment will not affect binding of nuclear factors to SP-1, CRE or c/EBP motifs in the human TNF promoter, while binding activity of NFκB in nuclear extracts is reduced to constitutive levels. This PDTC treatment effectively prevented the rise in transcript levels and it almost completely blocked synthesis of TNF protein. A similar blockade of TNF transcript levels was observed in PCR analysis of PDTC traeted blood monocytes. The data support the idea that NFκB is central to expression of the human TNF gene in monocytes and they suggest that substances like PDTC may be useful to control detrimental effects of TNF.

EXPRESSION OF LBP- AND CD14-mRNA IN THE HUMAN HEPATOMA CELL LINE HepG2

F. Stelter, U. Grunwald, H. Dietz, K. Vaczi, M. Ehlers, C. Krüger, C. Schütt
Dept. Med. Immunology, Ernst-Moritz-Arndt-University, Greifswald, Germany

The human hepatoma cell line HepG2 was cultured under serum free conditions in the presence of LPS (E.coli 055:B5, 100 ng/ml) and/or hu rIL6 (>40 U/ml).

The inducibility of CD14 and LBP expression was analysed by PCR and protein analysis. We found that the cells were able to express CD14- as well as LBP-mRNA constitutively. Whereas the level of CD14 mRNA did not change after stimulation with LPS and/or IL6 the level of LBP-mRNA increased after stimulation with IL6. It was not possible to detect membrane bound CD14 on the cell surface by FACS analysis or soluble CD14 in the culture supernatant by ELISA technique. LBP concentrations were measured by a newly developed functional assay using FACS-analysis of LPS-FITC binding to CD14. IL6 was able to induce LBP release into the supernatant, whereas LPS did not influence the cells. The IL6 inducing capacity could be enhanced by simultaneous addition of LPS.

CONSTITUTIVE NUCLEAR NFκB IN CELLS OF THE MONOCYTE LINEAGE.

M. Ströbel, T. Sternsdorf, A. Pforte, B. Passlick, P.A. Bäuerle, H.W.L. Ziegler-Heitbrock. Institute for Immunology, University of Munich, MPI for Biochemistry, Martinsried

The pleiotropic nuclear factor NFκB is involved in the expression of cytokines, of cell surface receptors and of viruses in human monocytes. Binding activity of NFκB can be detected in monocytes as well as in the monocytic cell line Mono Mac 6 without intentional stimulation, even under serum free and LPS free conditions, as demonstrated by gel shift analysis of nuclear extracts. Such constitutive NFκB can be detected in several cell lines of the myelomonocytic lineage, but not in Molt 4 T-cells or K562 stem cells. The amount of LPS-induced NFκB appears to be enhanced with differentiation, but the constitutive NFκB was not increased in the more mature cell lines, like Mono Mac 6, even after treatment with vitamin D3. A variable expression of constitutive NFκB was detected in primary blood monocytes and several tissue macrophages independent on the stage of differentiation. The data show that cells of the monocyte system under conditions that exclude major external signals do show constitutive NFκB without an apparent correlation to the stage of differentiation.

EXPRESSION OF SURFACE MARKERS ON ALVEOLAR MACROPHAGES (AM) FROM PATIENTS WITH HIV-INFECTION OR SARCOIDOSIS AS DETECTED BY FLOW CYTOMETRY

M. Subklewe, K. Wassermann, E. Schell-Frederick
I/III Medizinische Klinik, Haus 11, Joseph Stelzmann Str. 9,
D-5000 Köln 41, Germany

The goal of this study is to detect and quantify surface antigens on human alveolar macrophages by flow cytometry. Expression of surface molecules has been shown to be associated with the functional capacity of these cells. The primary antibodies were selected to measure antigen presenting capacity (HLA-DP, DQ, DR), monocyte-like cells (Leu M3, Leu M5, My7, My9) and the state of cell activation (Transferrin-R, Leu 15, 27E10, RM 3/1, IL-2R, ICAM 1). FITC-labeled F(ab')2 anti-Ig served as a second antibody. A CD 2, 3, 19 cocktail was used to gate out lymphocytes. The results are expressed as the median linear fluorescent intensity of the test antibody divided by that of the isotype control. This quotient indicates the intensity of specific antigen expression and corrects for variation in cell autofluorescence between patients. To date we have analysed cells from 30 HIV-infected patients, 10 patients with newly diagnosed sarcoidosis and 13 normal controls. The results show significantly increased intensity of Leu M3, Leu M5, Leu 15 and HLA-DP expression in both patient groups. In contrast, there is significantly higher expression of Transferrin-R in sarcoidosis as compared to controls but no increase in AM from HIV-patients.

MACROPHAGE DIFFERENTIATION IN MACROPHAGE COLONY STIMULATING FACTOR-DEFICIENT MICE FOR THE OSTEOPETROTIC (*op*) MUTATION.

Kiyoshi Takahashi, Makoto Naito, Yuki Morioka, Shuji Umeda, and Leonard D. Shultz.
Second Department of Pathology, Kumamoto University School of Medicine, Kumamoto, Japan, and the Jackson Laboratory, Bar Harbor, Maine, USA

In mice homozygous for *op* mutation (*op/op* mice), this mutation results in a defect in the coding region of M-CSF gene, leading to a total absence of functional activity of macrophage colony stimulating factor (M-CSF). In the mutant mice, serious deficiencies of monocytes in peripheral blood, monocyte-derived macrophages, splenic marginal zone macrophages, and osteoclasts were observed. In many tissues, numbers of macrophages variably decreased, particularly in the ovaries and uterus. However, numerical reduction of macrophages was not prominent in the spleen and brain. These *op* macrophages were small, round, and immature. Ultrastructurally, they showed poor development of intracellular organelles, particularly lysosomal compartments, and few cytoplasmic projections. In the *op/op* mice, serum GM-CSF level was higher than in the normal littermates. In co-culture of normal mouse bone marrow cells on a fibroblast cell line established from an *op/op* mouse, they stopped differentiating into macrophages at the stage of monocytes. However, less than 5% of immature macrophages were detected, corresponding to the *op* macrophages. In culture, a major cytokine secreted by the *op* fibroblast cell line was demonstrated to be GM-CSF. Compared to macrophages developed in cultures with GM-CSF, M-CSF, or IL-3 respectively, GM-CSF-derived macrophages closely resemble the *op* macrophages. All these results suggest that GM-CSF mainly supports the differentiation of macrophages in *op/op* mice and that the *op* macrophages are M-CSF-independent macrophages derived not from monocytes.

THE ROLE OF MEDIATORS IN THE PATHOGENESIS OF SILICOSIS. I. STIMULATION OF CELL PROLIFERATION OF HUMAN PNEUMOCYTES TYPE II (LINE A-549) INDUCED BY SUPERNATANTS OF QUARTZ DUST EXPOSED HUMAN MACROPHAGES

Ursula Thiel, B.Jung, N.H.Seemayer, Helga Idel
Medical Institute of Environmental Hygiene at the University of Düsseldorf, Gurlittstr.53, D-4000 Düsseldorf, F.R.G.

Silicosis is a pulmonary disease caused by quartz containing dusts resulting in lung fibrosis.
In pathogenesis of silicosis macrophages play a pivotal role.
Human marophages were obtained by cultivation and differentiation of human monocytes from the peripheral blood. Macrophages were incubated for 24 hours with Dörentruper crystal quartz flour (grinding no.12, particle size smaller than 5µm) at a non-toxic concentration. Thereafter supernatants were collected.
In earlier studies we found, that supernatants of quartz dust treated human macrophages in culture lead to remarkable cell proliferation of human lung fibroblasts (Wi-38).
By addition of a "competence factor" (plateled derived growth factor) stimulating effect of the cell proliferation factor was further enhanced.
These results suggest that the cell proliferation factor belongs to growth factors of the "progression type". The factor which was provisionally designated as "fibroblast proliferation factor" is characterized by a relative thermostability (56°C, 1 hour).
Now we investigated the effect of supernatants on human pneumocytes type II cells (line A-549). After addition of the supernatants initially spindle shaped pneumocytes were detected, followed by epithelial-like cells when cell proliferation progressed.
Induction of spindle-shaped pneumocytes type II cells could also be seen after addition of pure tumor necrosis factor alpha (TNFα). However, in this case no cell proliferation was observed.
Results indicate that supernatants contain at least two mediators: the tumor necrosis factor alpha and a proliferation factor.

LIPID A PARTIAL STRUCTURES: INHIBITION OF LPS-INDUCED MONOKINE PRODUCTION. A.J.Ulmer[1], W.Feist[1], T.Kirikae[2], F.Kirikae[2], H.Heine[1], S.Kusumoto[3], T.Kusama[1], H.Brade[2], U.Schade[2], E.Th.Rietschel[2], and H.-D.Flad[1]. [1]Dept.of Immunol.and Cell Biol., and [2]Dept.of Immunochem.and Biochem.Microbiol., Forschungsinstitut Borstel, Borstel, Germany, [3]Dept.of Chemistry, Osaka University, Osaka, Japan, [4]Daichi Pharmaceutical Co. Ltd., Tokyo, Japan.
Lipopolysaccharide (LPS) from the cell wall of gram-negative bacteria is responsible for a variety of pathophysiologic events (e.g. fever, septic shock) during infection. These events are predominantly mediated by monokines (IL-1, IL-6, and TNF) produced by the infected host. LPS consists of a hydrophilic polysaccharide and a covalently linked hydrophobic lipid part, termed lipid A. Lipid A represents the endotoxic principle of LPS, i.e. the biological effects of LPS are reproduced by free lipid A. The successful chemical synthesis of lipid A and corresponding partial structures of LPS, such as *Escherichia coli*-type lipid A (compound 506 or LA-15-PP) and precursor Ia (compound 406 or LA-14-PP) has provided the experimental basis to investigate the bioactive regions of LPS with regard to structure-activity relationships. A structure-dependent hierarchy of LPS and LPS partial structures with respect to their IL-1-, IL-6-, and TNF-inducing capacity was demonstrated, showing that the hexaacyl type lipid A LA-15-PP is able to induce monokine production by human monocytes, while the tetraacyl compound LA-14-PP exhibited no inducing capacity. The synthetic LA-14-PP and its phosphonooxyethyl analogue PE-4 became of particular interest since our studies show that LA-14-PP is able to block LPS-induced monokine production by human monocytes in a specific manner. In order to achieve a better understanding concerning the molecular basis of this inhibition, we have investigated whether LA-14-PP and other synthetic lipid A partial structures (LA-15-PP, LA-22-PP, LA-23-PP, LA-24-PP, and PE-4) are able to influence the binding of LPS to monocytes/macrophages. When comparing the inhibition of binding of ^{125}I-LPS to the inhibition of biological activity we found that both, LA-14-PP as well as PE-4, are the best inhibitors of LPS-binding to human monocytes as well as preventors of monokine production tested. Taken together, our results provide strong evidence for the concept that inhibition of LPS-cell interaction by LA-14-PP and other lipid A partial structures is based on a competitive inhibition of a specific LPS-binding protein of the responder cell. In this way these compounds may be able to prevent the fatal endotoxin-induced reactions of an infected host.

SOLUBLE CYTOKINE RECEPTORS AND THE TREATMENT OF INFLAMMATION.

David L. Urdal. Immunex Corporation, 51 University Street, Seattle, Washington 98101.

Cytokines are proteins responsible for the regulation of the hematopoietic cells responsible for the maintenance of the immune system. Two cytokines which participate in the process of inflammation are Interleukin 1 (IL-1) and tumor necrosis factor (TNF). The receptors to these cytokines have been cloned and naturally occurring soluble isoforms of these receptors can be detected in physiological fluids, which has lead to speculation that soluble receptors may help to regulate the cytokine response. Experiments *in vitro* and *in vivo* have demonstrated that recombinant soluble IL-1 receptor and TNF receptor bind IL-1 and TNF with high affinity and that soluble receptors are effective at neutralizing the toxic consequences of IL-1 and TNF in animal models. Given the increasing evidence that IL-1 and TNF play important roles in mediating a variety of acute and chronic inflammatory states of clinical concern, the clinical development of recombinant soluble IL-1 receptor and TNF receptor in the treatment of diseases such as allergy, septic shock, arthritis and graft versus host disease has been aggressively pursued. The results of animal toxicology and pharmacology studies and human clinical studies will be discussed.

ACTION OF PICHILAN ON NITRITE PRODUCTION BY A LONG-TERM-CULTURED RESIDENT MACROPHAGE LINE

N. Vallot (1), F. Boudard (1), C. Cabaner (1), P. Poindron (2), M. Bastide (1)
(1)Laboratoire d'Immunologie, Faculté de Pharmacie, Montpellier, France
(2)Université Louis Pasteur, Centre de Recherches Pharmaceutiques, Département d'Immunologie, Immunopharmacologie et Pathologie, Illkirch, France

Our aim was to study the action of pichilan, a (1 -> 3)-ß-D-glucan isolated from the cell wall of *Pichia fermentans* (CBS 187), on a murine macrophage cell line MALU obtained from lung explants of C57Bl / 6 lpr/lpr mice. Previous studies in our laboratory showed that pichilan has an immunostimulating effect on murine macrophages; exposure of macrophages to the glucan leads to increased cytotoxicity against bacteria. We investigated here some of the mecanisms underlying the action of pichilan. Macrophages can exert their microbicidal activity through two metabolic pathways: production of reactive oxygen intermediates (ROI) and production of reactive nitrogen intermediates (RNI). We measured the production of ROI and RNI by chemiluminescence and colorimetry (Griess reaction), respectively. The cells were cultured in 75-cm^2 flasks in RPMI 1640 medium supplemented with 10% fetal calf serum. We tested different extracts of glucan (FP 42, 45-46, 47, 48 and 50) on luminol-amplified zymosan-induced chemiluminescence. FP 50 caused the strongest production of superoxide anion production (ROI).We then tested the effect of FP 50 on nitrite production by the Griess method (RNI). The macrophages were plated at 1 x 10^6 cells / ml of culture medium per well in 24-well multititer plates and the liberation of nitrite was evaluated by incubating the macrophages with glucan and / or lipopolysaccharide (LPS). Each test was carried out in triplicate. FP 50 was tested at different final concentrations: high (0.03, 0.05, 0.07 and 0.1 mg / ml) and low (0.002, 0.004, 0.006, 0.008 and 0.01 mg / ml). A kinetic study (24, 48, 72, 96, 120 and 144 hours) was also performed. Under our experimental conditions, the production of RNI was statistically significant after incubation for 72 h with the glucan at concentrations between 0.002 to 0.01 mg / ml ($P < 0.05$). A linear relationship between the amount of nitrite produced and the incubation period was observed for concentrations from 0.002 to 0.03 mg / ml. The low concentrations seemed to be more effective on nitric oxide production, but these results have to be confirmed. Pichilan at 0.01 mg / ml induced the most significant liberation of nitrite (control: 4.633 ± 1.109; FP 50 at 0.01 mg / ml: 9.4 ± 1.687 µM NO_2^- after incubation.for 72 h $P < 0.05$). Furthermore, production was inversely proportional to the concentration of pichilan. After activation with LPS (100 ng / ml: final concentration), the macrophages were able to produce nitrite, a combination of LPS and glucan induced increased production (control: 3.4 ± 0.2; FP 50 at 0.01 mg / ml: 8.750 ± 0.350; LPS at 100 ng / ml: 15.45 ± 0.450; FP 50 + LPS: 18 ± 1.3 µM NO_2^- after incubation for 72 h $P < 0.01$) .Repeated treatment with glucan did not increase nitrite production compared with the single treatment. Our results suggest that the bactericidal activity of pichilan on murine macrophages can probably be explained by the ability of the glucan to induce reactive nitrogen intermediates.

IDENTIFICATION AND CHARACTERIZATION OF MONOCYTE CHEMOTACTIC PROTEINS OF THE IL-8 FAMILY

By Jo Van Damme, Paul Proost, Jean-Pierre Lenaerts, René Conings and Ghislain Opdenakker
From the Rega Institute for Medical Research, University of Leuven, B-3000 Leuven, Belgium

In response to infection, phagocytes are attracted to the inflammatory focus through the generation of chemotactic gradients. Recently, chemotactic factors belonging to a novel family of proinflammatory proteins (chemokines) have been identified. In contrast to the classical chemoattractants (e.g. C5a, FMLP) these molecules specifically affect the migration of single types of leukocytes. Within this family of structurally related low Mr factors, interleukin-8 (IL-8) is a well characterized neutrophil activating protein. IL-8 can be grouped into a class (designated CXC-chemokines) based upon the position of the two NH_2-terminal, conserved cysteines. Monocyte chemotactic protein-1 (MCP-1) belongs to a second class (CC-chemokines) in which these cysteines are adjacent. MCP-1 is an attractant for monocytes but not for neutrophils. Except for some platelet products, these inflammatory proteins can be induced in various cell types (fibroblasts, endothelial cells, monocytes, lymphocytes) in response to a variety of stimuli, including cytokines.

Cytokine-stimulated human tumor cell lines secrete several related chemotactic factors including IL-8 and MCP-1. We describe the isolation and characterization of two novel monocyte chemotactic factors from MG-63 osteosarcoma cells. Although these proteins copurified with MCP-1 and IL-8 on heparin-Sepharose, they could be separated by cation-exchange FPLC and reverse-phase HPLC. The corresponding 7,5 kD and 11 kD proteins were NH_2-terminally blocked but were identified by sequencing peptide fragments. They showed a primary structure mostly related to that of MCP-1 and were therefore designated MCP-2 and MCP-3, respectively. MCP-2 and MCP-3 are also functionally related to MCP-1 because they specifically attract monocytes, but not neutrophils *in vitro*. The chemotactic potency (specific activity) was comparable for all three MCPs. Intradermal injection of these proteins in rabbits resulted in selective monocyte recruitment *in vivo*.

MRP14 IS A MAJOR PHOSPHATE ACCEPTOR IN HUMAN MONOCYTES

Christian van den Bos and Clemens Sorg
Institute of Exp. Dermatologie, von-Esmarch-Strasse 56, W-4400 Münster, FRG

MRP14 is a calcium-binding protein assigned to the S-100 protein family and is expressed during differentiation of myelomonocytic cells; it is also abundant in infiltrating monocytes during inflammatory processes. It has been described to exist in phosphorylated forms, the function of this modification, however, is to date unknown.

Here, we attempt to evaluate the significance of MRP14 phosphorylation.

In order to analyse the process of MRP14 phosphorylation we employed a two-dimensional electrophoresis system consisting of isoelectric focussing and SDS-PAGE in the first and in the second dimension, respectively. Proteins were blotted onto membranes for further analysis.

The two-dimensional protein blots were then analysed threefold. First, by autoradiography to determine the amount of phosphate incorporated into MRP14 and other proteins, second, by general protein staining to estimate the quantitative distribution of proteins and third, after removal of the general protein staining, by immunostaining to identify MRP14 isoforms. This procedure allows for a high degree of comparability.

As a result of the immunostaining, we could identify six MRP14 isoforms with an apparent molecular weight of 14 kDa, five of wich were major spots. By densitrometric scanning we assessed the quantitative distribution amongst the five dominant MRP14 isoforms as being 16, 16, 17, 17 and 35 percent. The results of the autoradiography were twofold. First, only two out of six detected MRP14 isoforms appeared to be phosphorylated. Since they were the major MRP14 isoforms, they accounted for approximately half of the detected MRP14. Second, MRP14 was a, if not the, major phosphate acceptor as compared with other cellular proteins. Further evidence for this derived from the general protein staining which indicated the high level of phosphorylation not being caused by quantitative dominance of MRP14.

The significance of this might be outlined as follows: If phosphorylation of MRP14 is to regulate function(s) of MRP14, then this phosphorylation has to be controlled with great sensitivity. This, however, requires high rates of phosphorylation, which we have demonstrated here.

APOPTOSIS IN TNF-α DEPENDENT MONOCYTE MEDIATED LEUKEMIC CELL DEATH. A MORPHOLOGICAL, FUNCTIONAL AND FLOW CYTOMETRIC ANALYSIS.

A.A. van de Loosdrecht, G.J. Ossenkoppele, R.H.J. Beelen[1], M.G. Broekhoven, M.M.A.C Langenhuijsen.
Departments of Hematology and Cell Biology[1], Free University Hospital, De Boelelaan 1117, 1081 HV, Amsterdam, The Netherlands.

Little is known about the precise mechanisms of monocyte mediated cytotoxicity. Using highly purified (countercurrent centrifugal elutriation) and interferon-γactivated human monocytes (10^2 U/mL, 24 hours) we have studied cell and cytokine mediated cytotoxicity against U937 cells, a human histiocytic lymphoma cell line. At an effector to target cell ratio of 10, monocyte mediated cytolysis of 82% ± 5 after 24 hours incubation could be observed which could be partially blocked by neutralizing anti-bodies to TNF, whereas monocyte derived supernatant mediated cytostasis could be fully reversed (colorimetric MTT-cytotoxicity assay). Light and electron microscopic examination showed the characteristic features of apoptosis of U937 cells after incubation with either monocytes or rhTNF-α. No signs of necrosis could be observed. The rhTNF-α induced apoptosis (10^4 U/mL) as measured by flow cytometry (hypotonic propidium iodide solution) paralleled the functional decrease in cellular viability (MTT-assay) of 20% ± 3 after 24 hours up to a maximum of 50% ± 4 after 48 hours. Actinomycine-D (0.025-2.5 nM) and Cycloheximide (0.2-20 nM) showed a dose dependent synergistic actvity with TNF-α, whereas EDTA (0.1-1 mM) did not show any inhibitory activity of TNF-α induced apoptosis. In contrast, quantification of apoptosis by flow cytometry of monocyte mediated cytotoxicity was lower as compared to the percentage of monocyte mediated cytotoxicity as measured functionally in the MTT-assay. Moreover, morphologically monocytes showed a highly phagocytosing activity with apoptotic bodies in phagolysosomes which may have led to underestimation of flow cytometric quantification of apoptosis. In conclusion, these data provide evidence that apoptosis is the major mode of TNF-α dependent monocyte mediated leukemic cell death. Furthermore, we adapted a method to quantify cytokine and cellular induced apoptosis of leukemic cells by flowcytometry.

LINEAGE SPECIFIC SUSCEPTIBILITY TO HUMAN MONOCYTE MEDIATED CYTOTOXICITY IN ACUTE MYELOID LEUKEMIA.

A.A. van de Loosdrecht, G.J. Ossenkoppele, R.H.J. Beelen[1], M.G. Broekhoven, M.M.A.C. Langenhuijsen.
Departments of Hematology and Cell Biology[1], Free University Hospital, De Boelelaan 1117, 1081 HV, Amsterdam, The Netherlands.

In view of cellular adoptive immunotherapy with cytotoxic monocytes we have studied human monocyte mediated cytotoxicity (MMC) against a variety of human leukemic cell lines and leukemic blasts obtained from patients with acute myeloid leukemia (AML). Highly purified and interferon-γ(IFN) activated human monocytes were incubated for 24-96 hours at different effector to target cell ratios (E/T). MMC was evaluated in a MTT-colorimetric cell-mediated cytotoxicity assay. TNF-α sensitive U937 cells (monoblasts) were highly susceptible (>90%) to MMC whereas TNF-α resistant HL60 cells (promyelocytes) showed a low susceptibility (10-50%). After differentiation induction of HL60 cells into a monocytic direction with $1.25(OH)_2D_3$ these cells became intermediately sensitive (50-90%), although these cells remain TNF-α resistant. In contrast KG1 cells (myeloblastic; TNF-α resistant) were fully resistant to MMC and at E/T >1 were induced to a higher proliferation rate. Leukemic blast cells from patients with AML showed a similar differential susceptibility to MMC depending on their myeloid or monocytoid origin according to the FAB-classification of AML. M1 cells (myeloblasts) were induced to proliferation, M2/M4 cells (myeloid/myelo-monocytic) showed no or a low susceptibility to non-activated MMC whereas M5 cells (monocytic) were intermediately to highly susceptible. After simultaneous incubation with IFN-γleukemic cells showed an increased susceptibility. These differences in susceptibility to MMC paralleled differences in responses to TNF-α, IFN-γand IL-3/GM-CSF (CSFs). M1-M4 cells were promoted to proliferate in the presence of CSFs whereas M5 cells did not show any response to CSFs. Furthermore, TNF-α served as growth factor for M1 cells and some M2 samples. In the presence of IFN-γ, TNF-α showed a highly cytolytic effect on M4/M5 cells. In conclusion, these data provide evidence that the differential susceptibility of leukemic cells to human monocytes may be related to their lineage specific origin. These differences paralleled a differential response to TNF-α, IFN-γ and CSFs. These data may have implications to select patients for adoptive immunotherapy with cytotoxic monocytes in AML.

ROLE OF MACROPHAGES IN THE RESISTANCE AGAINST TRYPANOSOMES

P. Vincendeau, S. Daulouède, M. Letocard, V. Neaud.
Laboratoire de Parasitologie, Laboratoire des interactions cellulaires
Université de Bordeaux II, Bat. 3A, 3ème étage, 33076 Bordeaux Cedex, France.

Macrophages play a key role in the control of protozoan parasites. In this study, the roles of macrophages in the resistance against *Trypanosoma musculi*, a natural parasite of the mouse and *T. brucei gambiense*, the causative agent of human sleeping sickness, were investigated. As the importance of the L-arginine : NO metabolic pathway has been described in the antimicrobial function of activated macrophages, the participation of reactive nitrogen oxides was also investigated .

Murine peritoneal macrophages from the 10th day of *T. musculi* infection were activated (H_2O_2 production, Ia expression, endocytosis), produced nitrite and, unlike resident macrophages, did not favor *in vitro* parasite multiplication. This cytostatic effect was suppressed by addition of N^G monomethyl-L-arginine (NMMA), an inhibitor of NO synthase. *In vitro* resident peritoneal macrophages activated with IFN-γ + LPS exerted a cytostatic effect on *T. musculi* which was blocked by NMMA. Treatment with authentic NO gas inhibited the proliferation of *T. musculi*.

Compared to the parasite multiplication observed *in vitro* in presence of Kupffer cells from normal mice, a trypanostatic effect was also observed in co-cultures of trypanosomes with Kupffer cells from *T. musculi*- or BCG-infected mice.

Human blood monocytes were cultured in vitro for 7 days before addition of *T. brucei gambiense*. A trypanostatic effect was observed when monocytes were activated by supernatants of lymphocyte cultures.

Use of neutralizing antibodies directed to cytokines to inhibit the properties of lymphocyte supernatants and use of recombinant cytokines to activate monocytes *in vitro* are in progress to clarify the mechanism of human macrophage trypanostatic activity.

HIV-INDUCED SYNCYTIA FORMATION IN HUMAN MONOCYTES/MACROPHAGES: A MICROCINEMATOGRAPHIC STUDY

H. von Briesen[1], U. Sander[2], K.-H. Seack[2], M. Kreutz[3], K. Becker[1], S. Müller[1], H. Rübsamen-Waigmann[1], R. Andreesen[3]

1) Georg-Speyer-Haus, Paul-Ehrlich-Str. 42-44, 6000 Frankfurt/M. (Germany)
2) Institut für den Wissenschaftlichen Film, Nonnenstieg 72, 3400 Göttingen (Germany)
3) Medizinische Klinik I, Hämatologie/Onkologie, Franz-Josef-Strauß-Allee 11, 8400 Regensburg (Germany)

To investigate the consequences of HIV infection in primary human monocytes/macrophages (MO/MAC) we have established a culture system where MO/MAC were grown on hydrophobic Teflon membranes. After *in vitro* infection with the monocytotropic HIV-1 isolate D117III the virus replicates to high titre in MO/MAC. The maximum virus production is reached between day 20 and 30 and remains at a high level over several weeks. No cell death is obseverved but the induction of multinucleated giant cells. Syncytia containing 50 to 100 nuclei with a diameter of 200 to 400 μm are found in HIV-infected MO/MAC cultures. The aim of this study was to follow the process of giant cell formation by microcinematographic methods. Therefore, cultures were monitored microscopically by time lapse cinematography with 35 mm films. A speed of shooting of 1 frame per second to 30 frames per hour resulted in visualization of cell movement at an 25 fold to 3,000 fold accelerated speed. The evaluation of the processed film revealed three morphologically and kinetically distinct MO/MAC populations: large round-shaped, sessil types with only slow motion (type A), large moving types with variable shape which cover long distances (type B), and small agile types which are very actively and rapidely moving throughout the cultures (type C). In non-infected cultures we very rarely found spontaneous fusion processes between MO/MAC, and in some cases we could demonstrate endomitosis. Hence, only few cells (<15%) with more than one nucleus were found. In HIV-infected MO/MAC cultures numerous cell fusions were demonstrated between the sessil MAC type (A) and the agile MAC type (C). Frequently, this process took place polarly at one site of the type A MAC. During a later phase fusions also between two existing multinucleated syncytia were seen. The entire process from single-nucleus stage to a multinucleated giant cell could be perceived.

This film documents *in vitro* the cytopathological formation of HIV-induced giant MO/MAC which can be found *in vivo* in microglial nodules of AIDS patients' brain.

The Georg-Speyer-Haus is supported by the Bundesministerium für Gesundheit and the Hessische Ministerium für Wissenschaft und Kunst.

ACTIVATION OF IRON RESPONSIVE ELEMENT BINDING PROTEIN (IRE-BP) BY 7,8-DIHYDRONEOPTERIN IN HUMAN MONOCYTIC CELLS

Weiss G, Doppler W, Hentze MW*, Werner-Felmayer G, Fuchs D, Wachter H
Institute for Medical Chemistry and Biochemistry, University of Innsbruck, A-6020 Innsbruck, Austria. *) European Molecular Biology Laboratory, D-6900 Heidelberg, Germany.

Intracellular iron metabolism is regulated at the level of mRNA stability and translation of iron storage and transport proteins mRNA by the interaction of a specific trans-acting cytoplasmatic protein, iron responsive element binding protein (IRE-BP), with a cis-acting RNA motif, called IRE, identified on 5'ferritin mRNA and 3'transferrin receptor mRNA. Low intracellular concentrations of low molecular weight iron cause activation and binding of IRE-BP to the IRE which results in reduced ferritin translation and increased transferrin-receptor mRNA stability and translation et vice versa. We investigated the influence of neopterin and 7,8-dihydroneopterin on IRE/IRE-BP interactions in this human monocytic cell line with characteristics of macrophages (THP-1). Cells were cultered in RPMI containing 10 % FCS, supplemented with medium, iron (100 µM final concentration), deferrioxamine (200 µM), neopterin, 7,8-dihydroneopterin (50 µM each), 2,6-diamino-hydroxy-pyrimidine (5 mM) or interferon-gamma (500 U/mL) for 24 hours and cell extracts were prepared by using the detergent Triton X-100. In parallel, a ^{32}P-labelled oligonucleotide, identically with the IRE, was synthesized in vitro according to the method of Milligan et al. (NAR, 15:8783;1987). Cell extracts were incubated with the ^{32}P-labelled IRE and binding of the IRE-BP to the IRE was analyzed by mobility shift assays. As previously shown, extracts from cells pretreated with iron showed low IRE-BP binding activity to the IRE, while administration of the iron chelator desferrioxamine resulted in increase of IRE/IRE-BP interaction. IRE-BP activity was also increased after administation of 7,8-dihydroneopterin, while it was not influenced by neopterin. Concomitant administration of iron and 7,8-dihydroneopterin also increased IRE/IRE-BP interactions, thus reversing the inactivating effect of iron on IRE-BP. Stimulation of cells with IFN-gamma resulted in formation of extremely high concentrations of 7,8-dihydroneopterin and in addition activation of IRE-BP could be observed. When cells were stimulated with IFN-gamma in the presence of 2,6-diamino-hydroxy-pyrimidine, an inhibitor of 7,8-dihydroneopterin synthesis, pteridine formation as well as IRE/IRE-BP interaction were drastically reduced. We conclude that dihydroneopterin may activate IRE-BP by reducing cysteine residues, which was shown to be of major importance for increasing IRE-BP affinity.

TNF-α-INDUCED MHC CLASS II ANTIGEN EXPRESSION IS INHIBITED BY IFN-γ ON THE MONOCYTIC U937-SUBLINE C119/9.

Martin Willheim, Alois Gessl, Andreas Spittler, Zsolt Szépfalusi, Hermine Agis, Othmar Förster, and Georg Boltz-Nitulescu.
Department of General and Experimental Pathology, Neubau AKH, Währinger Gürtel 18-20, 1090 Wien, Austria

IFN-γ has been shown to increase the expression of class II antigens in a variety of cell types. We report the establishing of a subclone of the monocytic cell line U937, termed C119/9. In contrast to U937 cells, on C119/9 only TNF-α can induce HLA-DR and partially -DP molecules. The strong effects of TNF-α (% of HLA-DR-bearing cells increases from 5 to 90, mean fluorescence intensity from 6 to 266) can be inhibited almost completely with IFN-γ. The effects of TNF-α and IFN-γ seems to be restricted to HLA-DR and -DP expression, whereas HLA-DQ is induced neither by TNF-α nor by IFN-γ.Preincubation of the cells with IFN-γ does not enhance its inhibitory effect, pretreatment with TNF-α up to 24 h shows that addition of IFN-γ blocks the TNF-α-triggered HLA-DR expression. Other surface antigens, like MHC class I molecules, FcγRI and FcεRII are upregulated by TNF-α and IFN-γ. Interestingly, various other cytokines which have been reported to be involved in MHC class II regulation, such as IL-4, GM-CSF, TGF-β and IFN-α are also able to suppress the TNF-induced MHC class II expression on C119/9. Furthermore, IL-6, which shares some regulatory effects with IFN-γ on monocytic cell lines, also inhibits the effects of TNF-α on MHC class II expression. Downregulation of MHC class II molecules by IFN-γ has only been reported in some experiments with B-cells, where it inhibits the action of IL-4. C119/9 cells clearly show monocytic features, e.g. they can be induced to differentiate upon 1,25-dihydroxyvitamin D3-treatment (induction of CD14, ability to reduce NBT). This aberrant form of U937 cells may be useful to study the regulatory mechanisms of cytokine-induced MHC class II antigen expression.

ANTAGONISTIC EFFECTS BETWEEN ENDOGENOUS INTERFERON-ß(IFN-ß) AND INTERLEUKIN 4 (IL-4) IN MOUSE MACROPHAGES

Zawatzky, R. and Nickolaus, P.
Angewandte Tumorvirologie, Deutsches Krebsforschungszentrum Heidelberg,
and
Falk, W.
Innere Medizin I, Klinikum, Universität Regensburg

IL-4 was initially described as a T_H cell factor based on its ability to enhance proliferation in stimulated B lymphocytes. Lateron, it was recognized that IL-4 had important effects on other non-lymphoid cells involved in the regulation of the immune response. In cultures of mouse bone marrow cells, IL-4 was reported to inhibit growth stimulated by IL-3 but to enhance colony formation in response to M-CSF. Moreover, similar to IFN-γ, IL-4 is able to induce tumoricidal activity and antigen-presenting capacity in mouse macrophages. Interestingly, however, IL-4 can also block the secretion as well as some biological effects of IFN-γ in human cells and recently, an inhibitory effect on the development of the IFN-induced antiviral state in mouse L-929 cells was also attributed to IL-4.
In cultures of mouse bone marrow derived macrophages (BMM), we have therefore studied possible antagonistic effects between IFN-α/ß and IL-4. Culture of bone marrow cells in the presence of M-CSF plus IL-4 completely inhibited the biological effects of the endogenous IFN-ß constitutively secreted by these cells. Macrophages became highly permissive to virus infection and induction of the IFN-responsive enzyme 2'-5' oligo-adenylat-synthetase (OASE) was inhibited on RNA and protein level. IL-4 treatment, however, proved ineffective in inhibiting the biological effects of exogenously added IFN-α. These results prompted us to investigate the effect of IL-4 on the expression of endogenous IFN-ß in BMM. Therefore, a PCR-based semiquantitative analysis of IFN-ß mRNA was developed. Using an IFN-ß reference cDNA harboring a deletion within the sequence to be amplified, we detected 5-10 IFN-ß but no IFN-α transcripts per 100ng of total RNA from M-CSF cultured BMM. IL-4 treatment, however, inhibited the appearance of IFN-ß transcripts in BMM. This observation points out to a specific physiological effect of IL-4 on the expression of endogenous IFN-ß in macrophages since virus-induced IFN gene expression was not affected in IL-4 treated BMM.

GANGLIOSIDES SUPPRESS TNF PRODUCTION IN HUMAN MONOCYTES

H.W.L. Ziegler-Heitbrock*, E. Käfferlein*, M. Ströbel+, C. Weber+, D. Flieger*.
*Institute for Immunology, +Institut für Prophylaxe der Kreislauferkrankungen, University of Munich, 8000 München, Germany

Both normal and malignant cells contain gangliosides as important cell membrane constituents, which, after being shed, may influence cells of the immune system. We have studied the impact of gangliosides on the expression of TNF in blood monocytes and in the monocytic cell line Mono Mac 6. While under standard culture conditions, bovine brain gangliosides (100 µg/ml) suppressed LPS stimulated TNF production fivefold in peripheral blood mononuclear cells (PBMC) and tenfold in Mono Mac 6 cells, suppression was more efficient under serumfree conditions. Purified gangliosides GD3, GD1a, GM3, GM2, and GM1 (10 µg/ml) were all effective in reducing TNF production in PBMC and in Mono Mac 6 by factor 10 to 50. Gangliosides appear to act at an early step of activation in that TNF transcripts were reduced and the mobilization of the nuclear factor NFκB was blocked. Furthermore, in time kinetics, gangliosides were effective for up to 30 min after addition of LPS. Gangliosides also blocked TNF-production induced by staphylococci and by Paf, but phorbolester-induced O_2^- production was not affected. The data indicate that gangliosides can specifically prevent activation of the TNF gene at an early step of signalling.

REGULATION OF CD14 IN THE MONO MAC 6 CELL LINE: H.W.L. Ziegler-Heitbrock[1], W. Schraut[1], P. Wendelgaß[1], M. Ströbel[1], T. Sternsdorf[1], M. Ehlers[2], C. Schütt[2], J.G. Haas[3]. [1]Institute for Immunology, University of Munich, [2]Dep. Med. Immunology, University Greifswald, Germany. [3]Dep. Mol. Biol., Massachusetts General Hospital, Boston, MA. USA.

The human monocytic cell line Mono Mac 6 expresses substantial amounts of CD14 as assessed by staining with the My4 antibody (86% positive cells). Treatment with LPS, PGE_2 or TPA will induce further maturation as evidenced by enhanced phagocytosis and expression of mCSF-receptor mRNA. LPS and PGE_2 will enhance cell surface staining with a more than twofold increase in antigen density and with a maximum effect at day 2. Furthermore, both reagents will increase soluble CD14 (sCD14) in the supernatant of Mono Mac 6 by factor 8-12. This effect appears to be transcriptionally controlled, since LPS and PGE_2, both enhanced the constitutive level of CD14 mRNA 6 to 9-fold. By contrast, treatment with TPA reduces cell surface staining of CD14, it does not induce sCD14 and there is a transient downregulation of CD14 mRNA. These data show CD14 expression in Mono Mac 6 cells can be differentially affected by different inducers of maturation.

THE NOVEL SUBSET OF $CD14^+/CD16^+$ BLOOD MONOCYTES EXHIBITS FEATURES OF TISSUE MACROPHAGES: H.W.L. Ziegler-Heitbrock, G. Fingerle, M. Ströbel, W. Schraut, F. Stelter, C. Schütt, B. Passlick, A. Pforte. Institute for Immunology, Dept. Surgery, Dep. Internal Medicine, University of Munich, Dep. Med. Immunology, University Greifswald.

The $CD14^+/CD16^+$ cells in human peripheral blood account for about 10 % of all monocytes in apparently healthy donors. These cells, when compared to the regular ($CD14^{++}/CD16^-$) monocytes, show a low expression of the CD14 antigen and a high expresion of the CD16 antigen. These differenences appear to be transcriptionally regulated as evident from concomitant changes in transcript levels as assessed by PCR. In 3-color-immunofluorescence, the $CD14^+/CD16^+$ cells exhibit twofold higher levels for class II, while CD11b and CD33 antigens are twofold decreased. Alveolar macrophages (AM) appear to be similar to the $CD14^+/CD16^+$ cells, since they also express higher levels of class II and lower levels of CD11b and CD33 when compared to the regular monocytes. Finally, monocyte-derived macrophages, obtained by 5 d culture of mononuclear cells in 10 % human serum, will develop low CD14 and high CD16 and they also upregulate class II and downregulate CD11b and CD33. Taken together, our data demonstrate features of mature macrophages in the novel subset of $CD14^+/CD16^+$ blood monocytes.

Author Index

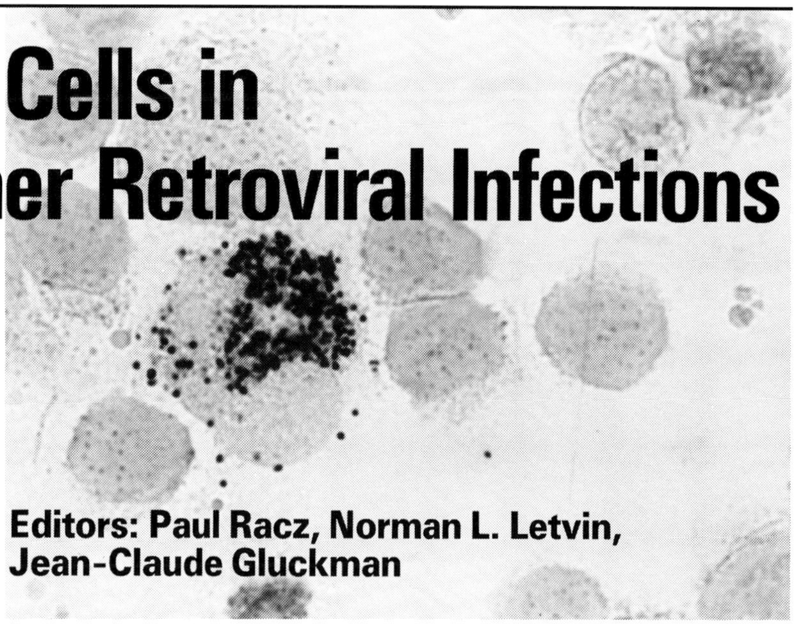